Less Than Crazy

Less Than Crazy

Living Fully with
Bipolar II

Karla Dougherty

Foreword by A. Carlos Altamura, M.D.

Da Capo
LIFE
LONG

A Member of the Perseus Books Group

Designed by Trish Wilkinson
Set in 12-point Adobe Caslon by the Perseus Books Group

Library of Congress Cataloging-in-Publication Data

Dougherty, Karla.
    Less than crazy : living fully with Bipolar II / by Karla Dougherty ; foreword by A. Carlos Altamura. — 1st ed.
        p.   cm.
    Includes bibliographical references (p.   ) and index.
    ISBN 978-1-60094-047-7 (alk. paper)
    1. Manic-depressive illness—Popular works. I. Title.
RC516.D68 2008
616.89'5—dc22   2008024908

First Da Capo Press edition 2008

Published by Da Capo Press
A Member of the Perseus Books Group
www.dacapopress.com

Da Capo Press books are available at special discounts for bulk purchases in the U.S. by corporations, institutions, and other organizations. For more information, please contact the Special Markets Department at the Perseus Books Group, 2300 Chestnut Street, Suite 200, Philadelphia, PA 19103, or call (800) 810-4145, ext. 5000, or e-mail special.markets @perseusbooks.com.

10 9 8 7 6 5 4 3 2 1

To the memory of
Debbie Geller.
It was much too soon.

Acknowledgments

IF IT WEREN'T for the profound kindness, generosity, support, and, oh yes, the patience of the people I love, this book would never have been written. First and foremost, thank you to my husband. DJ, you have always been there for me: "In you, I have life's promise." Thank you to my family of friends, including Frances Pelzman Liscio, whose goodness never ceases to amaze me and whose talent graces the drawings in this book; Betsy Elias, who somehow found the time to go through the manuscript painstakingly and find what I'd missed; Stefanie Nagorka, whose unwavering friendship kept me on the straight and narrow; and Marilyn and Lance Garcy, whose astonishing selflessness enabled me to keep going.

The talented professionals at Da Capo have me in awe, including my editor, Katie McHugh, and Renee Caputo and Connie Day. Thank you all.

James Welch, M.D., has been remarkable, not only as a psychiatrist but also as an editor. And I owe special thanks to Rose Oosting, Ph.D.: this book would not have been written without you.

Thank you to my agent and friend Joelle Delburgo, who has always believed in my abilities.

And a big thank you to my goddaughter, Michelle Shang, just because.

Contents

PART THREE
How Is Bipolar II Treated — and How Can I Live Happily?

Foreword

For a long time, no distinction was made among different types of bipolar disorder. Either you were bipolar or you were not. Unfortunately, this "all or nothing" approach to the disorder created many misconceptions about the disease and resulted in its being broadly associated with schizophrenia and borderline personality disorder. Today, however, we know there is a "bipolar spectrum," where bipolar I (characterized by frequent co-morbidity with more serious emotional disorders) appears at one end of the spectrum, and where milder, less debilitating bipolar diseases appear the further along the spectrum one goes.

Bipolar II is a much milder form of bipolar disease. Yes, there are contrasting swings of exuberance and depression, but they manifest themselves in "quieter" ways; mania usually exhibits as anxiety, and depression often exhibits as a milder and more atypical form of depression. It is this subtlety of symptoms—which can still strongly affect quality of life—that makes bipolar II so difficult to diagnose.

One of the more relevant characteristics of bipolar II is anxiety, encompassing a range of forms from panic attacks to social anxiety and obsessive-compulsive symptoms. Because of these links to anxiety, bipolar II is often overlooked and misdiagnosed.

People have asked me what makes a person who is diagnosed with bipolar II different from someone who is anxious. It's human nature to be anxious before a big event, before a presentation, or in a new job or relationship. But whereas this "natural" anxiety dissipates after the event or presentation is over, or as the job becomes familiar or the relationship more solid, anxiety in bipolar II not only lingers but gets stronger with each day.

Many of my patients worry about imaginary crimes and are persistently anxious about something they did or said that has no bearing on the actual reality. They often "read" facial expressions wrong, seeing something negative in people where it doesn't exist. This anxiety builds up . . . until, usually within a week or so, the patient plummets into a depression. The anxiety is still there, combined now with feelings of hopelessness and helplessness.

It is at this stage where most people with bipolar II come for help, and where the misdiagnosis usually takes place. A physician sees a person who is depressed—and prescribes an antidepressant that not only will not work but also can create mania.

As director of the Depressive Disorders Treatment Center in Milan, Italy, I have seen many bipolar II patients who initially came in for depression or anxiety. I have learned to read the signs of this condition—the hypomania, the heightened anxiety, the debilitating depression that won't go away. But when such a patient is given the right medication (be it Lithium, an anticonvulsant, or an antipsychotic such as quetiapine), I have seen the lingering depression quickly subside, allowing the person in pain to regain his or her life.

As a professor of psychiatry at the University of Milan as well, I have also had the privilege of conducting studies on various medications for bipolar disorder, among them the quetiapine (brand name: Seroqeul) mentioned above. I've long worked on research about antianxiety medications and their potential for abuse. People with bipolar disorder often have addictive personalities, and unfortunately, the antianxiety medications play right into this vulnerability to addiction. Even worse, the patient needs more and more of the medication as he or she builds up a tolerance. It also creates extreme fatigue and a cognitive "fogginess." But we found that quetiapine, taken in much smaller doses than with schizophrenia or bipolar I, has a calming effect, just like an antianxiety medication, but without affecting cognitive abilities or causing fatigue. And most important, quetiapine is not habit-forming. The results of a four-year follow-up of patients on quetiapine therapy have just been published in the *Journal of Affective Disorders* (March 2008),[1] and I am happy to report that low amounts of quetiapine were as effective in keeping major depression and mania at bay as were older, more traditional therapies, such as lithium bicarbonate, at higher doses.

Europeans have known about bipolar II for over a decade. In fact, it is twice as common as bipolar I within the population. Studies such as the Netherlands Institute of Mental Health Survey and Incidence Study (NEMESIS) and the EPIDEP in France found distinct differences between people with bipolar I and those with II. Those with bipolar II showed symptoms earlier in life; their depression was more chronic; they were more apt to take risks when in a hypomanic state; and, as I wrote in the *Journal of Affective Disorders* in 2007, they are more prone to substance abuse and anxiety—from panic disorder to social phobias, generalized anxiety disorder, and obsessive-compulsive disorder. They are also more inclined to succumb to alcoholism or become addicted to drugs. Because the disease is usually not diagnosed for, on average, ten years, it makes sense that people afflicted with bipolar II usually have a poor quality of life.

With this book, Karla Dougherty attempts to solve the "mystery" of bipolar II. It is a thorough, informative, and moving account of what it ultimately means to have the disorder. I know it is her hope, as it is mine, that *Less Than Crazy* will find an audience among people who have lived "half-lives," who have grappled with their symptoms for years, who have always blamed themselves for their transgressions, and who have felt intense shame, guilt, and misunderstanding for much too long a time. It will also be of great help and interest to family members and friends of individuals with bipolar II, as well as an invaluable source of information for readers who simply want to understand this condition better.

This book is yet another reason to hope that psychiatric disorders, such as bipolar disorder and depression, will continue to lose their stigma, and that more and more people will seek out help and, quite simply, get well.

A. Carlos Altamura, M.D.
Milan, Italy

Introduction
Giving a Name to Your Pain: It's Real

I NEVER THOUGHT I'd write this book. Although I've collaborated on over forty published books, this one was so personal that I was afraid I'd be embarrassed, found out, ostracized. I mean, bipolar disorder? The doctor who told me I had bipolar also told me it was the "minor" kind, bipolar II. But in my head, when I first heard the news, all I heard was *bipolar disorder,* a diagnosis that for me seemed synonymous with borderline personality disorder (as in stalking and plopping bunnies in a pot) or, worse, schizophrenia (as in "really crazy"). In my "now labeled crazy" mind, this doctor was telling me I was insane.

Yes, I got depressed—maybe even really depressed, but that was countered with days or weeks when I had so much nervous energy I wished I could bottle it for later, to draw on during those days or weeks when I felt like a sea slug. So, sure, something wasn't right with me. I was fearful, a little paranoid, and a whole lot of anxious. I would accept depression, even a clinical one. I'd accept an anxiety disorder, social or otherwise. But bipolar???

I silently promised myself that there was no way in hell anyone would know that I was given this diagnosis (which I still wasn't sure I had). It would be my secret, shared with only my therapist, my husband, and a few close friends.

And then something happened. I started taking the *right* medicine for the disease and I started to feel better. In fact, I felt better than I had in forty years. I was beginning to heal from a condition that had me locked up in solitary so long that I didn't even realize how deprived and miserable I'd been. During those years, it was as if I were being severely punished for a crime I not only didn't commit but didn't even know existed.

Over the next few months, as I continued to feel better, I started telling a few more people. And no one gasped. No one turned away in horror. In truth, every time I mentioned my condition and emphasized the "type II," people didn't know what I was talking about; they were more curious than shocked. What's bipolar II? Like me, they knew only about bipolar disorder, manic-depression, mood swings.

That got me thinking. If it took me forty long years to be diagnosed, how long did it take other people? And what about the ones who haven't yet been diagnosed? The ones who don't have full-blown, black American Express card episodes, but who are never able to, quite simply, feel good—about anything?

And that's when I realized that I not only wanted to write this book, I *needed* to write this book. The more I learned about bipolar II, the more I realized that my assumptions about bipolar—and mental health conditions in general—had been wrong. I needed to make the world see bipolar disorder not, as many people do, as some crazy label, but as a very real disease that can be treated. Even more important, I needed to reach other misdiagnosed people who had bipolar type II, so they wouldn't have to wander around for forty years in their own makeshift desert. I wanted to tell these people that, no, they weren't "crazy." They had a disease, a mild form of bipolar disorder that, just like diabetes or arthritis, could be treated.

So that's why I wrote this book and why I called it *Less Than Crazy*.

My Story

Before I was diagnosed, I had bought into the unfortunately all too common stigma. I had assumed that bipolar disorder was something only "crazy" people had—so how could I have it? Nor did I recognize my symptoms as bipolar. I didn't plan grand trips to Paris with a bank account in the red. I didn't splurge on dozens of expensive shoes in a single spree (although I have been known to spend a tad more than I should on make-up). I wasn't the life of the party, the one you or anyone else wanted to meet. By the same token, I was never so depressed that I messed up my job, missed a deadline, or zoned out during a meeting. I could function just fine on a daily basis, thank you very much.

I thought all people with bipolar went to hospitals to "rest." I assumed they had scars on their wrists and anonymous boxes on the bookshelf filled with illicit drugs. I didn't do cocaine or drink myself unconscious. I never tried to kill myself, and I hadn't thought about it. (Okay, maybe when I was in tenth grade and the boy of my dreams broke up with me, or my best friends ganged up on me à la *Mean Girls*, or my parents were being impossibly stubborn and confining—i.e., not giving me permission to drive the family car—I would think about swallowing pills and leaving a note that would make everyone suffer with guilt for the rest of their natural lives. But those thoughts were usually accompanied by a Righteous Brothers song playing at full volume, many cigarettes near an open window, a bolted bedroom door, and an unmade bed.)

Suicide? Screaming out names? Irrational to the point of harm? No, no, no. I might be a little melodramatic, a little moody and hypersensitive, "down" on occasion, but that was it.

And yet. . . .

Living in Fear

There was always something nagging that stayed with me, this "extra" persona that even my superego couldn't control. I couldn't have been truly happy, not really, because I was always afraid of reaching for something I desired. Whether it was writing the novel people always thought I had the talent to pen, traveling to other countries, or going out with an incredibly sexy man . . . or whether it was simply asking for a drink, eating in a restaurant, standing up, hell, even talking—I worried about all of it, incessantly. I grew up near Manhattan and was actually afraid to get into a cab. I was always thinking that *this driver is going to hurt me* and then *who will take care of my dog* and *none of this matters anyway because I'm going to be fired, lose all my money, and live in a car.* I always settled for security because I lived in fear. After all, if I felt secure, I wouldn't worry as much, right? Wrong.

I tried, I really did. I'd pop a tranquilizer and go to work, ready to face the folks I believed hated me. I'd go to a party trying for a mysterious aura—the unapproachable, confident *mademoiselle*—so I didn't have to meet someone (and maybe have them kill me on the way home after forcing me to have sex). I wouldn't dare contribute to a conversation. Instead, I'd wait for someone else to give an opinion, and then I'd say, "Yeah, me too." I was a perfect chameleon, a yes-person, the exception to the rule that "You can't please all of the people all of the time."

No one knew the turmoil that lurked just below my Chanel make-up. She didn't write a novel? Guess she really didn't want to. She's so nice to everyone? She has to be a phony. No one knew the conversations I had in my head or how miserable I was. If they did, I worried, they'd probably flee so fast they'd get that plane ticket to Paris before the thought even occurred to me (which it wouldn't because I wasn't bipolar).

Nor did anyone have any idea of the struggles I endured each morning when I got up. It took a huge amount of courage to push away the covers along with the anxiety that, apparently, had been the way my mania showed its face.

Yes, anxiety. Of course, everyone gets anxious sometimes. But I'm not talking anxious before the SATs, or before your wedding, or on the first day of a new job. I'm talking anxiety that was like a giant hand constantly poking me in the side.

Anxiety was always there as my shadow companion. Throughout my life, it was ready to slam the door shut when I wanted to go outside to play; when I went to college and had the chance to fall in love with someone exciting; when I wanted to stay single and live in Manhattan. It rushed me home to ensure I didn't leave the stove on, heckled me as I worried that my friends didn't like me, and cried exaggerated tears when I felt guilty about something no one even remembered. Later on, it pushed me to accept piles of hack writing assignments instead of writing the novel that was in my heart.

It didn't stop, but it stopped me. At any given moment I was sure I would get lost in the car, in the subway, in the airport. I would be kidnapped while taking a cab, waiting for a bus, or just walking down the street. I would fall off my bicycle and become paralyzed, hitting the concrete and becoming brain-damaged. I would get fired. I would get Alzheimer's. I'd gain weight, eat too much, not fit in, lose my looks, lose my friends, lose my dogs. Lose.

All my worries were equal. They multiplied and came together like one of those balls of rubber bands, growing bigger and bigger with each new fear.

To say I was exhausted all the time is an understatement. I was overwhelmed by my mind, and my body couldn't keep up. Worse, most of my anxieties, so real to me, were like the voices schizophrenics hear: they *weren't* real. They were usually so off the mark that the idea of trusting my intuition would be akin to writing a suicide note.

I worked hard at staving off the anxiety with years of therapy and antianxiety medication. Insight after insight, chemical after chemical attacked my fears with some degree of clarity and reinforcement. But the antianxiety treatment never lasted. And it was never enough.

Coping

My only defense was an offense: I became hypervigilant, watching people react to something I said. I analyzed the way they expressed themselves, the way they looked. Was that a sneer? Whoops. I'd better change that line of thought. Did they hate the movie? Better tell them I did, too. My energy went into pleasing others. Like Woody Allen's *Zelig,* I became a mirror where people could see themselves reflected in a positive light— and allow me to bask in their afterglow.

Why? Because, over the years, the one way I learned to master my anxiety was by believing everyone liked me and that all was in order in my world. The slightest raised eyebrow, the possible wrong behavior, and, boom, the whole thing would fall apart and I'd become even more anxious.

But if everyone liked me, my anxiety could subside. It became my goal.

Obviously, this stance was impossible to sustain. My problem was that despite my best efforts, I couldn't hold on to it for even a day. My need to be loved was like Chinese food. An hour later and I needed to hear it again.

Eventually, my maniacal (with the emphasis on "mania") anxiety would become so exhausting that I'd swing the other way. I wouldn't become less anxious, but I would abandon my hyper-vigilance. Instead of trying to gauge the world around me, I made my world my bed. Like a soldier who'd been on guard duty for too many double-shifts, I literally collapsed.

I might have dreamed about becoming a famous novelist, an actress, or a world traveler, but my reality aspired to a much more modest goal: I just wanted to be calm.

Misdiagnosis

By chance, about twenty-five years ago, I discovered that I had a knack for translating complicated medical jargon into everyday language. I wrote one book on post-traumatic shock disorder anonymously for a physician who specialized in the condition, and soon after, I began writing more books on medical subjects for the general public. It was an ideal career move: I was able to hide behind someone else, letting his or her words reach people while I was safe from anxiety-creating scrutiny. And because I had learned early in my life to be accommodating, I was able to capture the voices of these authorities in exactly the way they wanted. Forget my novel, my early promise as a writer in my own right. Instead, I became a ghostwriter for other people in the health care field.

Ironically, I'd written four books about the brain by the time my bipolar II was diagnosed. I could recite information on the lobes of the brain, the different sections of the brain, and what functions each serves. I must have used the computer analogy and the corporate analogy to describe the different areas of the brain and their specific functions more times than I could count. I knew how each area of the brain interacts with every other and with the rest of the body, as well as how messages travel through the brain.

In my research and writing, I'd covered the gamut of mental illness, writing about clinical depression, chronic depression, masked depression, obsessive-compulsive disorder, attention-deficit hyperactivity disorder, conduct disorder, panic attacks, math phobia, school phobia, social phobia, eating disorders, borderline personality disorder, schizophrenia, substance abuse, generalized anxiety disorder, learning disabilities, thyroid disease, and low blood sugar. I'd even written about manic-depression.

Through them all, I never had a clue about my own condition.

Why? Because none of the medication, none of the billable hours, and none of the self-help books were treating the core of what was wrong with me: bipolar disorder, more specifically bipolar II. The depression part was easy. But anxiety as mania? The toe-tapping, nail-gnawing, prism-thinking, lip-biting, worrying, worrying, worrying, jumping out of my skin? Mania? No wonder it took so long to get the right diagnosis!

The Reality of Bipolar II

I wasn't alone in my early beliefs about bipolar disorder. Most people believe manic-depression is synonymous with insanity.

They often see it as the disorder that drives the artist. It was manic-depression that compelled Van Gogh to cut off his ear, that made Sylvia Plath put her head in the oven, that led Ernest Hemingway to put a gun to his head. And, indeed, they are partially right. Manic-depression, or bipolar I, is a serious mental illness that, when left untreated, can destroy lives, both literally and figuratively.

A less dramatic "version" of bipolar disorder, bipolar II, is a relatively new diagnosis that has been recognized in Europe for at least a decade but has only been studied in the United States for the past few years. Officially, having bipolar II is defined as having had one or more major depressive episodes and one or more hypomanic episodes. I call it the *milquetoast* version of manic-depression, a disease in which a person, when in a manic cycle, is crippled by anxiety, irritability, and highs just bold enough to be embarrassing. Unlike the bipolar I sufferer who might buy out an entire department store, a person with bipolar II might spend hours trying to figure out what to wear. Instead of being the life of the party, a person with bipolar II might be too nervous to go to the party at all. And unlike the bipolar I sufferer who might attempt suicide when in the throes of a depressive cycle, a person with bipolar II might be incapacitated by guilt over an imaginary crime.

Does bipolar II sound similar to depression? Does it sound like an anxiety or obsessive-compulsive disorder? Yes—and these are two of the main reasons why it isn't yet on every doctor's radar screen. The majority of physicians, psychiatrists, and psychologists will call it depression and prescribe an antidepressant. Or they may say the patient has generalized anxiety disorder (GAD) and prescribe a tranquilizer. Or perhaps they'll call it a depression combined with symptoms of anxiety or conduct disorder or ADHD or any number of other disorders, and leave it at that. Unfortunately, antidepressants alone won't work. Neither will antianxiety drugs. Bipolar II is a lifetime condition that requires the correct treatment, or the individual is very unlikely ever to get better. Without the proper diagnosis, a person suffering from bipolar II will continue to live a half-life fraught with anxiety, bitterness, and unresolved potential.

This might not sound terribly alarming, because, one might wonder, how many people really suffer from a disease that carries a whiff of manic-depression? The statistics are actually quite surprising: a 2003 nationwide survey conducted by the University of Texas Medical Center in Galveston found that *approximately nine million Americans,* or 4 percent of the population, suffer from bipolar II.[1] Only two years earlier, in 2001, a survey undertaken by the National Depressive and Manic-Depressive Association (DMDA) put the number at 2.5 million Americans.[2] The results of these two surveys indicate that the number of Americans *known* to be suffering from this disorder had almost tripled in only two years!

In addition, both surveys found that one-third, or 35 percent, of the people with bipolar disorder waited an average of ten years—*ten years*—to get help. Worse, when they finally did seek help, they were frequently misdiagnosed.

I was finally diagnosed after years of false turns. How many more of us are out there?

I have a confession. I wrote this book not just altruistically, to let the world know about bipolar II; I also wrote this book because I was tired of suffering alone. I wanted to find others who also felt alone, strange, during the years they lived with a misdiagnosis. I wanted to interview them and see how their symptoms cropped up. I wanted to start a dialogue, a community where we'd be able to support each other, to talk about our disease without the threat of laughter, annoyance, or "Is there a straitjacket in the house?" thinking.

Although in some cases the names have been changed, the stories in *Less Than Crazy: Living Fully with Bipolar II* are real, and you, the reader, may find their experiences resonant with your own. And you might find the courage, conviction, and hope you didn't know you had.

Do You Have Bipolar II?

If you, too, have been diagnosed with untreatable depression or chronic dysthymia (a low-grade depression where you're never quite happy, where things aren't quite right); if you find yourself continually worried and anxious over, well, everything (including the fact that you're feeling good); if you find yourself angry and full of rage a lot of the time; if your emotions are right up there in your face, changing with the weather—then come on down! You may have undiagnosed bipolar II.

You too might suspect—along with your therapist and family— that you suffer from a serious or chronic mental disorder, or, if you haven't yet gone for help, that you are just plain miserable and unhappy, and that's just the way it is. Over the years, you too may have developed a keen sense of self-loathing. You may have thought of life as trying to scale a brick wall: climbing a fair distance, but eventually losing your grip and falling back to the ground.

Like myself and the other people I interviewed for this book, you might be nervous every time you leave the house; you might be working in a job that's below your potential but is "safe"—because the wider world is too terrifying to handle. You might always be cash-poor, confused, and plagued by problems maintaining a relationship. You might think happiness is some-thing for other people, other lives.

Like millions of people worldwide, you might think your problems are all your fault, when, in fact, your disease simply hasn't yet been properly identified and treated.

How to Use This Book

In this book, you'll find out whether your problems may indeed stem from bipolar II. And you may discover that your inability to finish a project is not laziness, that your anxiety about going out is not a weakness in your psyche, and that not pursuing your dreams is not the result of your lacking passion or desire but, instead, has a very real physical basis.

True, there are many facets to our personalities that we *do* cre-ate. Not everything can be attributed to bipolar II. But I know that once I was diagnosed (and got over the initial "Ohmigod, I *am* crazy" thoughts), the relief was profound. I could do good, intense, focused work. I could enjoy myself. I could spend days, and even months, not feeling that vague sense of foreboding that followed me like an evil shadow for decades. I could even find more order in my life: sticking with a diet and exercising two or three times a week. I was even balancing my checkbook every month.

I've divided *Less Than Crazy* into three parts. The first part explores what bipolar II is—how it's different from bipolar I, and its characteristics, including the definition of the new "buzzword" hypomania.

Part Two explores the "whys" of bipolar II—the different theories regarding its roots, the role of brain chemistry, its symptoms in both the depressive and the manic cycles, and its diagnosis.

Part Three discusses all-important treatment: from medicines to lifestyle changes, from holistic supplements to talk therapy and group support.

Throughout the book, you'll also learn more about me and hear the stories of other people who have finally had bipolar II correctly diagnosed. You'll read the results of studies, research articles, and clinical trials, as well as hear from authorities—clinicians, researchers, and psychiatrists—in the field to help you find self-knowledge, sound medical advice, and the personal strength of knowing you are not alone.

I hope this book helps you find some answers before another year goes by. I hope that in hearing the voices of people with this condition, and in reading the words of experts in the field, you will more easily discover that profound relief—and happiness—that it took me far too many years to find.

PART ONE

Do I Have Bipolar II — and How Does It Affect My Life?

1

A Disease in Its Own Right

Somehow, we view mental health as totally
under a person's control.

—Dr. James Pennebaker,
author and educator

Everybody has an opinion about bipolar disorder:

"She's really crazy. She's bipolar."

"He is so manic. It's going to come crashing down."

"She belongs in an institution, she's so manic-depressive."

"He was a mad genius, but he was manic-depressive."

"Who could live with her? She's crazy. Definitely bipolar."

"Of course, he's in the hospital. He's bipolar, isn't he?"

These words, and comments reflecting the misguided view that Dr. Pennebaker describes above, are remarks that I've overhead often—and, sadly, I'm not the only one who has heard them. The ill-informed attitudes they spring from have kept mental illness in the closet all these years. Bipolar disorder is as "crazy" as a heart condition, as "insane" as a broken foot. It's a disease, pure and simple. But because it affects our brains rather than our hearts, its symptoms are not as cut and dried. Behavior is not as black and white as a clogged artery or a high cholesterol ratio.

The Differences between Bipolar I and Bipolar II

Bipolar I

Classic bipolar I disorder, or manic-depressive illness, is characterized by extreme mood swings. During a manic episode, people with bipolar I may lose the need to sleep or eat; they may talk and think erratically and become easily angry and irritated. They may be delusional, thinking, for example, that they are having relationships with famous people, or they may become sexually promiscuous, or adopt a very grandiose attitude, claiming expertise in areas they know nothing about.

During a depressive episode, people with bipolar I have severe feelings of hopelessness and helplessness. They may be unable to get out of bed, yet ruminating thoughts prevent them from sleeping. They may not be able to work or have relationships. They can become very paranoid. At the worst, people with bipolar I may feel such dismay that they try to commit suicide.

According to the National Institutes of Mental Health (NIMH), the signs and symptoms of bipolar I include

A Manic Bipolar I Episode

- Increased energy, activity, and restlessness
- Excessively "high," overly good, euphoric mood
- Extreme irritability
- Racing thoughts and talking very fast, jumping from one idea to another

- Distractibility, can't concentrate well
- Little sleep needed
- Unrealistic beliefs in one's abilities and powers
- Poor judgment
- Spending sprees
- A lasting period of behavior that is different from usual
- Increased sex drive
- Abuse of drugs, particularly cocaine, alcohol, and sleeping medications
- Provocative, intrusive, or aggressive behavior
- Denial that anything is wrong

A manic episode is diagnosed if elevated mood occurs with three or more of these symptoms most of the day, nearly every day, for one week or longer.

A Depressive Bipolar I Episode

- Lasting sad, anxious, or empty mood
- Feelings of hopelessness or pessimism
- Feelings of guilt, worthlessness, or helplessness
- Loss of interest or pleasure in activities once enjoyed, including sex
- Decreased energy, a feeling of fatigue or of being "slowed down"
- Difficulty concentrating, remembering, or making decisions
- Restlessness or irritability
- Insomnia (or sleeping too much)
- Weight loss (or gain)
- Chronic pain or other persistent bodily symptoms that are not caused by physical illness or injury
- Thoughts of death or suicide, or suicide attempts

A depressive is diagnosed if five or more of these symptoms last most of the day, nearly every day, for a period of two weeks or longer.

Bipolar II

Bipolar II is different. It isn't as dramatic as bipolar I. Bipolar II lingers; it is chronic. Compared to classic manic-depression, its symptoms are more subtle—a humid, sultry summer night to the other's belligerent thunderstorm. Bipolar II has been referred to as "sunny" or "soft" bipolar, presumably in contrast to bipolar I's dark havoc. An individual can also be in the throes of "rapid cycling," in which the prevailing mood switches from one to the other within hours; can undergo "mixed cycling," in which she or he feels both "sunny" and "dark" at the same time; or, throwing out the word *bipolar* altogether, can experience DM, which stands for "mainly depression" (this condition is not known as MD, for obvious reasons).

People with bipolar II tend to experience anxiety to a greater extent than those with bipolar I (38 percent vs. 23.7 percent). In addition, people with bipolar II have more phobias (22.5 percent vs. 11.8 percent) and more depressive episodes, which is one of the reasons why it is often misdiagnosed as unipolar depression.[1]

Another problem faced by people with bipolar II—and the professionals who treat them—is confusion. Although the most recent research shows that the condition is indeed a distinct entity and a disease in its own right, many people still consider bipolar II a part of a bipolar spectrum disorder (BSD). This constitutes a broad range of bipolar disease, containing not only I and II, but *six* other types as well—making the condition sound more like a parody than a serious disorder that affects approximately 9 million Americans.

• THE BIPOLAR SPECTRUM

Type $^1/2$, schizobipolar: a combination of schizophrenia and bipolar disease

Type I, mania without depression

Type I$^1/2$, a preponderance of mild mania (hypomania) combined with depression Type II, a more balanced combination of hypomania and depression

Type II$^1/2$, depression paired with marked mood swings within the normal range (cyclothymia)

Type III, bipolar disorder created by antidepressants

Type III$^1/2$, bipolar disorder created by stimulants

Type IV, bipolar disorder born from a highly emotional temperament (hypothymic)[2]

Most studies fail to separate bipolar II from major depression but, rather, treat it as a component of major depression.[3] In fact, as wide a range as 25 percent to 65 percent of all patients diagnosed with major depression have been diagnosed in later, more in-depth interviews, as exhibiting bipolar II.[4]

Unfortunately, because bipolar II is a mood disorder, diagnosing it as depression often means that a person gets only half the medication he or she needs. Without mood stabilizers, treatment will probably be unsuccessful, create more frequent and intense manic episodes, or, at its very worse, lead to suicide. Studies suggest that many suicides that had been believed to be the tragic result of a major depression actually resulted from untreated bipolar II.[5]

The problem with bipolar II lies in its subtlety. People with the condition usually only seek help when they are in a depressive cycle. After all, why would anyone seek help when he or she feels confident, needs little sleep, has tremendous creative energy, and stands out in a crowd? Unfortunately, this initial manic "high on life" attitude sooner or later becomes anxiety, irritability, anger, and irrationality—symptoms seldom associated with mania but very much considered signs of depression.

Ironically, when a person with bipolar II actually does go into a depressive cycle, the symptoms are usually atypical, the very opposite of what one assumes depression is. Instead of a loss of appetite, there's compulsive and binge eating. Instead of insomnia, there's sleeping too much (hypersomnia). Instead of detachment from emotion, there is exaggerated vulnerability to feeling hurt when faced with rejection and criticism (interpersonal sensitivity). Instead of feeling better as the day goes on, as in most depressions, the individual feels progressively worse throughout the day.[6]

Given how its symptoms often mimic other conditions, it doesn't come as a surprise that bipolar II is often diagnosed only when nothing else is left. It's the diagnosis of last resort.

• BIPOLAR OVERSEAS

Numerous studies in Europe put the number of people with bipolar II at between 2 and 5 percent of the population; they have also found that it is twice as common as its more famous counterpart, bipolar I.[7] One study in particular, the Netherlands Institute of Mental Health Survey and Incidence Study (NEMESIS), revealed that people with bipolar disorder not only reported a poorer quality of life, but a quarter of them (25.5 percent) had never sought help for the emotional problems—not from their primary care doctor, from an alternative care professional, or even informally from their family or friends.[8]

The Official Characteristics of Bipolar II

Specific anecdotal behaviors are only one way a mental health professional may determine whether you have bipolar II. Consider the action and reactions described in the list of statements above more of a "jumping off point," a sign that, yes, the feelings and actions you are worried about are real.

Fortunately, bipolar II has received enough recognition in recent years to be included in the *Diagnostic and Statistical Manual of Mental Disorders,* Fourth Edition, Text Revision (DSM-IV-TR), the official updated sourcebook used by psychotherapists, psychiatrists, and other mental health professionals to pinpoint a mental illness, as well as to provide a diagnostic number that is useful for health insurance and Medicare purposes, peer study consistency, global categorizing, and selection among treatment regimens.

The DSM-IV-TR classifies bipolar II as a condition in which a patient exhibits one or more depressive episodes accompanied by at least one hypomanic episode. In addition, a person must never have had an outright, "break from reality" bipolar I manic episode; his or her moods must not be accounted for by schizophrenia, delusional disorder, or other psychotic disorders; and the symptoms must cause significant distress in daily life.[9]

Because symptoms are as arbitrary as perception, a skilled therapist uses not only the DSM-IV-TR to make a diagnosis, but also his or her insight, experience, and research. To that end, Figure 1-1 and Figure 1-2, respectively, list the manic and depressive symptoms of bipolar II culled from clinical trials and epidemiologic studies (research that surveys large populations).

• GENDER BIAS

Research shows that more women suffer from bipolar II than from bipolar I. They won't get severe mania, but they get depressed. They are also at higher risk for rapid cycling (more than four highs and lows in a year) and are harder to treat with standard regimens. Why? Possibly because of hormonal differences and psychosocial factors.[10]

FIGURE 1-1. Symptoms of Bipolar II in Manic Cycle[11]

Recurrent and lasting 1 to 3 days:

Anxiety (including separation anxiety)
Irregular sleep patterns
Less inhibited and shy
More talkative than usual
Impatience
Rapid shifts in mood (lability)
Easy irritability
Euphoria
Overconfidence
Heightened sensitivity to environment
Increased coffee and/or cigarette consumption
The "Overs": Over-activity, over-planning, energy overdrive
History of panic attacks
Substance abuse
Compulsive eating or bulimia
Increased sex drive
Phobic behavior (including agoraphobia and social phobia)
Obsessive-compulsive behavior (including intrusive thoughts)

Do You Have Bipolar II?

If you've picked up this book, chances are that you suspect something is wrong, that you don't go through your day like other people. Maybe you've been terribly sad . . . maybe you felt good on Tuesday, but by Friday you're feeling down. Maybe you have this anxiety that just won't go away. Or maybe the good feeling you have almost feels euphoric, as though you were high on drugs. Is that you? You could have bipolar II.

Look over the statements in Figure 1-3 and see whether any of them has applied to you consistently for more than four

FIGURE 1-2. Symptoms of Bipolar II in Depressive Cycle[12]

Early onset, recurrent, and lasting 3 to 6 months:

Abrupt onset (usually)

Hypersomnia (sleeping too much) (in most cases)

Weight gain (usually)

Self-pity

Somatization (the manic cycle's anxiety turned into physical problems)

Depressive feelings that are worse in the evening

Unrelenting jealousy

Suspicion and paranoia

Difficult, demanding behavior

Narcissistic misinterpretation of people's actions and words (called ideas of reference)

Slowing down of motor skills (psychomotor retardation)

Excessive feelings of guilt

Depersonalization (losing one's self-identity and sense of reality)

Withdrawal and isolation

Derealization (alterations in perception in which familiar things "feel strange")

Suicidal ideation (thoughts)

---

weeks. Remember that bipolar I is easier to see; it's the lead actor playing to the balcony. Bipolar II is more the chorus line; it's harder to differentiate, even harder to diagnose. A hypomanic or manic cycle can last as little as one day, but depression usually lasts from three to six months! (*Please note that nothing takes the place of your doctor's supervision. If any of these statements sounds like you, make an appointment to see your physician. Only he or she can tell you whether you have bipolar I or II, or any other disorder for that matter.*)

FIGURE 1-3. Do These Statements Sound Familiar?

1. Sometimes I feel exhilarated—I can literally do no wrong.
2. The exhilaration I feel never lasts. Before I know it, I'm down in the dumps.
3. I worry all the time.
4. I can't go to work unless I've taken a tranquilizer.
5. I can't go to sleep unless I've taken a tranquilizer.
6. Sometimes I think I have an obsessive-compulsive disorder. I think about the same things in my mind, over and over—and they usually involve my causing an imaginary slight, usually to another person. I'm reluctant to leave the house. I'm always thinking there's a pending disaster waiting to happen, especially when I'm happy. I've done antidepressants, antianxiety meds, talk therapy, even herbal supplements. Nothing does the trick.
7. I have trouble getting up in the morning. I don't want to face the day. But by nightfall, I'm wide awake and can't get to sleep.
8. I definitely "feed my feelings." I'm a mindless eater, and the more refined carbs the better.
9. I'm easily irritated and quick to anger.
10. I never voice my own opinion. If someone asks, "What movie do you want to see?" or "Where do you want to eat?" I'll always answer, "Whatever you want." I'd never make my own decision!
11. I'm like a see-saw. My moods go up and down, up and down, one or two times a day.
12. I'm hypersensitive.
13. I'm a woman and I get the most depressed around my period.
14. I need almost constant reassurance.
15. I don't feel centered; I'm not comfortable in my own skin.
16. I might be anxious, but I don't hear voices or hallucinate, and I live in the real world.
17. I can't focus on the job at hand.
18. Everybody likes me (at least I think so)—and I worked hard to make it that way.

continues

19. I never seem to climb out of debt, even when I try to budget.
20. I spend more money than I make.
21. I always reach for something bigger and better than anyone else—not because I'm competitive, but to prove (to myself) that I'm as good as they are.
22. My body is in constant motion; I fidget (jiggling legs, tapping fingers, biting my lip).
23. There's no grey area for me. Either I'm up or I'm down.
24. I've been to more therapists than I can count—and none of them have helped.
25. A doctor diagnosed me as having bipolar I and gave me lithium—which made me nauseated and bloated and didn't do a thing to help.
26. Antidepressants don't help my depression. If anything, they make me wired—and still depressed.

If you answered "yes" to more than twenty-one statements, it's possible you have bipolar II. In fact, if you answered "yes" to even just half (thirteen statements), it should send up a red flag. It's important to talk to a health care professional about your symptoms.

The Myths Surrounding Bipolar Disorder

Sometimes the hardest thing for us to do is face our problems head-on. This is especially true of a disease that carries such a stigma in our society. What makes this condition even more insidious is that it's diagnosed incorrectly more times than correctly. In fact, studies show that misdiagnosis is the most common characteristic of bipolar disorder.[13]

Not only is bipolar II difficult to diagnose in observing a person, but the myths that surround the disease compound the problem. Here are some of the more common ones that we can finally put to rest.

Myth 1: You can just snap out of it

If only. I spent years trying to do just that and then feeling even worse because nothing I did—scheduling, relaxing, sleeping, exercising, praying—worked. I chalked it up to my own fault that I would be anxious on vacation ("How could I be so spoiled!") or that I didn't write a novel ("Guess I didn't want it enough"). No, bipolar disorder is a real biological disease, with its own brain chemistry and even its own chromosome strands. In fact, many health insurance companies have taken bipolar disorder out of the mental health realm and are now calling bipolar an organic disease—which means the coverage available for its treatment is the same as that provided for a sore throat or a twisted ankle and is not contingent on the number of therapy sessions your health plan allows.

Myth 2: If you are bipolar, you're always swinging from up to down to up again

Although mood cycling can be rapid, most people with bipolar II tend to stay in a depressive state for a long time; their hypomanic episodes are more fleeting. Some people get stuck in a depression and stay there for years. The good feeling you have after a depression has lifted is *not* necessarily hypomania. And the older you get, the more time may elapse between pendulum swings. Some people can have long-term remission, where their symptoms are blessedly held at bay.

Myth 3: If you have bipolar II, you can easily slip into the more severe bipolar I

Wrong again. Although studies show that it can happen, it is more the exception than the rule. In a five-year time frame, only 5–15 percent of people with bipolar II slipped into bipolar I. You are more susceptible to mania if you mess up your sleep-wake cycle, such as when you travel between time zones, stay up to all hours to make that deadline, quiet your baby in the middle of the night, or have insomnia (which can be due to your anxiety!).

Myth 4: All I need is medication and I'll be stable

Studies show over and over again that treatment for any mental disorder requiring medication is much more effective when accompanied by some form of talk therapy. If you are afraid of the cost, speak to your health insurance company. Most of them have some form of mental health coverage.

Myth 5: If I let my employers know, they'll cook up some kind of reason to fire me

Here's some good news: We don't live in a Charles Dickens novel. We aren't trampled, forgotten, or pushed into a dungeon if we show any sign of mental illness. But unfortunately, yes, there is some risk in telling your boss, because she or he might become overly concerned, watching you more closely to ensure that you're working. And you might be treated differently by your colleagues. But you don't have to tell your employer. After all, would you tell your boss that you have cardiovascular disease or diabetes? Would it be something you *have* to "lay on the table"? No. The only time it can become an issue is if it begins to interfere with your work. Whether or not you tell your boss you have bipolar II is up to you. The Disability Discrimination Act (DDA), passed in 1995, makes it illegal for employers to discriminate against employees on the basis of any type of disability, and that includes mental conditions.

In today's business world, if you work efficiently, pitch in and perform your tasks, and use your skills to enhance the company, no one will care if you have bipolar II or six carbuncles sticking out of your neck. If you stop working efficiently or your mistakes start piling up, then sure, that decline in performance can become an issue. But then again, *anyone* whose mistakes start piling up is putting his or her job in jeopardy!

And remember: bipolar II is a mild form of bipolar disorder. In most cases, it *won't* impinge on your work life to the point of incapacitation. But if you find yourself out of sorts, if you find that your thinking is getting foggy and your work is getting sloppy, call in sick. It's not a lie—you are sick. It's just not in your chest or your stuffed up nose. If you need a day off because you're feeling very stressed out, taking a sick day or two won't hurt you— unless a crucial deadline is hanging in the balance. (And if the timing is awkward, call your doctor. He or she can adjust your medicine accordingly and set up additional therapy appointments. Also, when you begin to recognize the signs of bipolar II behavior creeping up, be sure to make time for self-care. Get to sleep early. Get a massage. Meditate. You can weather the storm even if you can't afford to take time off.)

Myth 6: Letting loved ones know I have bipolar II will negatively affect my relationships

Not if those relationships are good ones. Your bipolar II is a condition, yes, but it is as much a part of you as diabetes or heart disease. If you're honest with those around you, you might find some solid support and real understanding. They can help you determine your moods, if you are becoming manic or depressed. And, as observers, they may notice irrational or depressed behavior before you do.

When should you let the people in your life know? That's up to you. I wouldn't bring it up on a first date, but certainly if your relationship is going well and you've gone out several times, you'd want to bring it up. Don't make it a "life or death" situation; don't paint a bleak picture. Just tell the person that you have this condition but you are being treated. Plain and simple.

Be prepared for your loved ones not to believe you. When I first mentioned my disorder to my family, they scoffed. I was just being Karla; I was fine. Sure, I had my "quirks," but everyone does.

But that's okay. The people who love you will love you, even if they are skeptical about your condition. Believe it or not, although it might be a big deal to you, it won't necessarily be a big deal to anyone else!

If someone you are dating or some of your friends back off, let them. You wouldn't want to be in a relationship with them anyway. In the long run, how many relationships built on lies or omission survive? The answer is very few indeed.

Myth 7: So what if I'm manic—I love being manic!

The very definition of hypomania is euphoria. (See Chapter 2 for detailed information on hypomania.) Who doesn't want to feel euphoric about themselves, about life? Who doesn't want to feel so good that they'll stand on the rail of a ship and declare themselves "King of the World" (just not on the *Titanic*)? Unfortunately, bipolar II hypomania doesn't stick around forever, and eventually, you'll either have a major depressive episode or experience the bipolar II equivalent of mania—when anxiety and fear take over your life.

A diagnosis of bipolar II is not a death sentence. And bipolar II doesn't have to be the end of who you thought you were. It's a disorder, just like diabetes or chronic fatigue or arthritis. The more you understand your condition, the more effectively you'll be able to explain it to the people around you.

In the spirit of understanding bipolar II better, the next few chapters will describe in depth its signs and symptoms and diagnosis.

2

Hypomania Defined

That's the difference between me and the rest of the world. Happiness isn't good enough for me. I demand euphoria!

—*CALVIN AND HOBBES*

WHEN I WAS a child, barely six, I wanted to row a boat. Never mind that I'd never been in a rowboat before this particular day at summer camp. A counselor had taken me and two other campers out on the lake. As we sat in the boat, it looked as if she were dancing, her arms graceful arcs, the water rippling with applause. It didn't look hard. And I loved leaving behind the noise of the other kids chattering away, the swimming and splashing near the water's edge, the busy jumble of beach towels and rubber thongs and beige nose plugs and flowered bathing caps. The sounds, the sights, were diminished and safe and contained. And only just a few feet from shore.

My mind was probably made up over the tuna noodle casserole at dinner, but it wasn't until late that night that I realized with a sharp pang how much I wanted to row that boat. I *needed* to row that boat. And I *could* row that boat. Why not? I had watched the counselor. One oar in the water, then the other, one in, one out. Easy.

I quietly pushed away my wool blanket, pulled on my shorts and blouse and sneakers that lay in a heap on the floor, and opened the bug-stained screen door of our bungalow. I ran down the hill to the lake. Victory!

The boats were on the shore, looking, in the haze of the late summer moon, like shadowy cliffs. I could only find one oar, half-buried in the grass. It was enough.

The oar was heavier than I had thought when I watched two of them effortlessly cut the water that afternoon. Holding the one oar with both hands, I walked over to the boat and dropped it inside. One more step. I had to push the boat off the shore into the water and then jump in, just as I had seen the counselor do.

The lake barely murmured, dark blue, hints of white. I could hear sounds coming from the water. Fish. We were the only ones awake.

The water was cold, but I didn't care. I had a mission: get to the middle of the lake where the quiet would enfold me like nurturing arms. Using both hands, I pushed the oar and used it as leverage to slip out onto the lake.

It worked! I was floating! The weeds and the mud at the lake's bottom no longer brushed the boat. I was moving. I started to row, continuing to use the one oar, first on one side, then on the other.

But suddenly it was dark on the lake, much darker than it had been only moments before. Murky. The silence was no longer comforting; my ears felt heavy; I was alone and the world had changed. What had I done? I wanted to go back.

I rowed and rowed, but the one oar was pushing me in circles. I couldn't turn around; I couldn't turn the boat, it didn't want to go, there were monsters down there, deep, deep, waiting. I was facing the far side of the lake; I couldn't see the shore.

The water gulped beneath my boat. The stars shimmered in the water's reflection. I tried to push the oar down into the water to see how deep it was. Even though I was practically kneeling down, my waist over the edge, the oar couldn't touch bottom. It was that deep.

Monsters. I was going to drown. I would stay out here all night and drown and no one would know. I cried out, tentatively at first. The whisper echoed over the water. "Helppppp . . ." as if it were far away, and I was, and no one came. "Help!" I shouted, so much louder now I could see the water move. I dropped the oar in my confusion and lost it to the monster.

There was only one way, I was certain: I had to swim to shore. I had learned to swim only the summer before, but it was either that or die. I panicked. I couldn't breathe. I jumped into the water, sneakers and all. It felt like forever. My arms ached. The water was cold, and as my sneakers became wetter and wetter, they felt heavy. I shoved them off. And swam. I should have drowned but I didn't.

The fact that I had to have been much closer to shore than I'd imagined didn't cross my mind.

I was only six, and the only punishment I received was a lecture and a bad head cold. But as the years went by, I continued to get myself into all sorts of scrapes, fueled by intense exuberance. Ride a two-wheeled bike without training wheels? No problem—except for a broken arm. Do a final project for science class overnight? Easy—except for getting an incomplete. Rent that super-expensive apartment? Sure—except for the four jobs I had to hold down to pay for it every month. . . . And on and on, a lifelong pattern that began way before the midnight swim. I thought I could do anything, everything, and the everything I did was a big deal. I had no idea that this impulsivity and false courage were symptoms of something else. Neither did anyone in my family.

Hypomania: The New "Buzzword"

Some people call it the glory before the storm. Others call it euphoria, passion, or bursts of creativity and pray it stays forever. Lynda, one of the people I interviewed for this book, described it as "my summer romance. It was fabulous, fantastic, and it would always end in a few months." Whatever adjective or metaphor you use, the actual emotion and behaviors go by the name of hypomania: the one and only great scene in the drama of bipolar II.

Hypomania is "a minor manic state," and it is usually exhibited before mania. For many people with bipolar II, it is the only mania experienced. In a few hours, a few days, a few weeks, it will be supplanted by depression. For others, hypomania is the gateway to mania. My hypomania matured along with my body. Over the decades, the lake turned into school, friends, work, and marriage. But that feeling that I could do anything and everything remained. I had the energy of a machine. I'd work on projects the whole night through, without the benefit of anything stronger than coffee. I still remember the serenity I felt as the sun rose and the birds began their dawn chorus. I could literally feel the blood circulating throughout my body, my heart, my lungs, my belly: I was alive and it was glorious!

This intermittent self-confidence (I chose not to call it self-aggrandizement) got me dates with interesting men and attracted a wide circle of friends. Everyone wanted to be with me.

I was beautiful! I had a *joie de vivre* that no one else had. I was special. (I chose not to call it self-delusional.)

Eventually, choosing wasn't an option; my glorious feeling would dissipate like melted snow. Either my joy turned into anxiety or it sank into the earth. I would spend days in bed, looking at the ceiling, my mind racing: I had to work. The deadline was approaching. "I have to work. But I'm not." I would cancel plans and stay at home with my dog, watching TV and getting fat. I couldn't go outside, let alone on a date.

Or I'd become so depressed that my energy stalled, grinding to a halt. From being able to do anything, I went to being able to do . . . nothing.

My life would become that rowboat up the lake without a paddle. And this time, there was no way I'd make it to shore.

Hypomania vs. Euphoria

That's the trouble with hypomania. It doesn't last. You can run with it when you have it, accomplishing amazing feats of drive and ambition, partying it up 'til the early morning, but eventually you'll crash. If you have bipolar II, you may become even more manic (read: anxious) and feel your head will burst with the worry upon worry upon worry settling in like the guest who wouldn't leave. Or you'll crash, becoming so depressed that you hate yourself, you can't do anything, and, by the way, who were you to think you could?

Hypomania is insidious. It can look like euphoria, and often is; as the bipolar disorder pioneer Kay Redfield Jamison says in her book *Exuberance: The Passion For Life*,[1] without the high energy nothing would be accomplished. But unlike joy or exuberance, hypomania turns on a dime, not just making a person vulnerable, as Jamison mentions, but dealing destruction. Anxiety settles in, depression pushes down. Like the old saying "It was great while it lasted," hypomania is great—and then it's gone.

When you're exuberant, you ride the tide. You make things happen. You inspire change. But hypomania isn't as powerful. It can't lead because it doesn't have a vision—only a faulty perception. It's the small-town party versus Macy's Thanksgiving Day Parade.

And unlike normal feelings of joy, hypomania doesn't just go away, leaving behind happy memories. Instead of afterglow, there is a crash—of shame, of self-loathing, of sadness that shatters like broken glass.

Have You Ever Experienced Hypomania?

Needless to say, the controversy surrounding hypomania has encouraged many clinicians to assess and study hypomania and its characteristics. Professor Jules Angst, one of the most renowned clinicians who study hypomania, and his colleagues in Zurich, Paris, Luleâ, Sweden, and London devised a self-assessment tool to pinpoint hypomania in an outpatient setting. The multilingual hypomania checklist (HCL-32) has been tested internationally, and the researchers have identified two different types of hypomania:

Type 1: Active/elevated hypomania: You are full of energy and can multitask without a problem. Your mood is elevated and your thinking is crystal clear.

Type 2: Risk-taking/irritable hypomania: You get angry easily; you are impatient and stubborn. But you'll also take a lot of risks, and your creativity feels as if it has no bounds.

Dividing hypomania into these two groups has proved helpful for physicians in assessing their patients. By recognizing the different ways in which hypomania can manifest itself, they are better able to diagnose bipolar II correctly, rather than mistaking it for a major depressive disorder (MDD), which is one of the most common errors in bipolar II treatment. (Most people who have bipolar II go to the doctor only when they are depressed. Hence the physician often makes the diagnosis of depression instead of bipolar II.[2])

In Figure 2-1 is a portion of the HCL-32 published in the *Journal of Affective Disorders* in 2005. As the patient responding to this checklist, you answer "yes" or "no" to each statement. Other portions of the checklist examine your current state of mind, your family history, the reaction of others when you are in this state, and how hypomania affects your life.[3]

FIGURE 2-1: Hypomania/Mania Symptom Checklist (HCL-32)

1. I need less sleep
2. I feel more energetic and more active
3. I am more self-confident
4. I enjoy my work more
5. I am more sociable (make more phone calls, go out more)
6. I want to travel and/or do travel more
7. I tend to drive faster or take more risks when driving
8. I spend more money/too much money
9. I take more risks in my daily life (in my work and/or other activities)
10. I am physically more active (sport, etc.)
11. I plan more activities or projects
12. I have more ideas, I am more creative
13. I am less shy or inhibited
14. I wear more colorful and more extravagant clothes/make-up
15. I want to meet or actually do meet more people
16. I am more interested in sex, and/or have increased sexual desire

continues

FIGURE 2-1. *continued*

17. I am more flirtatious and/or am more sexually active
18. I talk more
19. I think faster
20. I make more jokes or puns when I am talking
21. I am more easily distracted
22. I engage in lots of new things
23. My thoughts jump from topic to topic
24. I do things more quickly and/or more easily
25. I am more impatient and/or get irritable more easily
26. I can be exhausting or irritating for others
27. I get into more quarrels
28. My mood is higher, more optimistic
29. I drink more coffee
30. I smoke more cigarettes
31. I drink more alcohol
32. I take more drugs (sedatives, antianxiety pills, stimulants . . .)

Excerpted from Angst J, Adolfsson R, Benazzi F, et al. The HCL-32: Towards a self-assessment tool for hypomanic symptoms in outpatients. *J Affect Disord*, 2005; 88: 217–233.

• HYPOMANIA: GOOD OR BAD? TALK AMONGST YOURSELVES

Is hypomania a part of bipolar disorder? Is it "manic lite," as John Mc-Manamy, author of *Living Well with Depression and Bipolar* and publisher of the e-newsletter *McMan's Depression and Bipolar Weekly*,[4] refers to it? Is it, as maintained by John D. Gartner, Ph.D., a clinical assistant psychiatrist at Johns Hopkins Medical School, and author of *The Hypomanic Edge: The Link Between (a Little) Craziness and (a Lot of) Success in America*, the vital temperament in our leaders that made our country great?[5] Or is it Kay Redfield Jamison's clinically understudied exuberance?

Many people with bipolar II believe that hypomania is their true personality, their un-bipolar self. In fact, medication may subdue these people too much, making them depressed and unable to function. Whether an illness, an episode, or a state of grace, hypomania feels good and, at least for me, doesn't feel bipolar at all. It's when the anxiety starts seeping in or the hopeless emotions start dragging you down that help is needed.

People who are pretty much in a hypomanic state all the time probably aren't reading this book. They're out doing things, being productive, living a full life. But if, like me before I got the right treatment, your hypomanic state is more of an episode, brief but beautiful, then read on. In the next chapter, you'll see how hypomania becomes a gateway to mania: a signal that something's happening to your psyche and it ultimately ain't good.

3

Swing High the Bipolar II Way
Anxiety

Early in life, I was visited by the bluebird of anxiety.
—WOODY ALLEN

RHONDA HAD NEVER bought anything from an infomercial—until now. The gizmo that did five kitchen chores in one got her by the time the announcer had shown only three. By the time he'd demonstrated how easy it was to clean, she was already calling the 800-number and giving her credit card information. She couldn't wait to get the product.

After a week, she started looking for the postal carrier, hoping the package was in that day's mail. When it finally came, she tore open the packaging, plugged it in, grabbed an apple, and . . . nothing. The machine was supposed to mince it in nanoseconds, but all it did was make a mess. Rhonda was furious, not only at the manufacturer's claims but also at herself for being "sucked in." She wrapped up the gadget and returned it. And that wasn't enough: she also e-mailed all her friends and family to warn them against the 5-in-1 kitchen miracle aid.

But a few days later, the anxiety set in. Rhonda was terrified that the manufacturer would find out that she'd been bad-mouthing the product. She was afraid they'd sue her (or worse!) for writing negative notes. She was so sure this would happen that she stayed up at night, unable to sleep. She even wrote new notes to everyone telling them that she was mistaken; it could have just been her own ineptitude. After a while, she was able to subdue her anxiety by putting herself down. But unfortunately, it was only a matter of time until something else would become the object of her "affect-ions."

––––––––

Lois was finally going on vacation. She'd been saving her money for over two years now in order to take her dream trip to Paris. Lois fantasized about meeting a sexy Parisian man; she saw herself sitting in an outdoor café, sipping coffee *au lait*. She organized everything for her trip a few weeks ahead of time, buying airline requirement bottles, guidebooks, the works. The biggest planning involved her poodle, Linus, whom she loved like her baby; she had been lucky enough to find a pet sitter who took care of him very responsibly when she went away for a weekend or a short trip, staying with him overnight in Lois's apartment. The pet sitter was wonderful; Lois would come home to a happy, healthy dog.

But she'd never gone overseas before—and this imposed a whole new set of worries. She met with the pet sitter a few days in advance and even had her come to the apartment right before she left so the dog wouldn't be alone. Lois wrote five pages of instructions and listed a whole host of emergency contacts. There was nothing else left to do.

But Lois had this nagging feeling; her heart would start to speed up and her mouth go dry. Was Linus okay?! Lois called the sitter from the airport, twice—both in the States and in France. All was well. When she arrived at her hotel, she called again. Each time she called the sitter, she felt enormous relief. Linus was fine. But by the next day, she was anxious again. She ended up calling the service every single day she was away. It didn't ruin her trip, but it sure came close. The sad thing was that Lois didn't have as much fun as she should have.

Roberta knew her bank account was running low; she balanced her checkbook herself. She also knew she wasn't getting paid for another week and a half. So she decided to budget, really budget: pastas, salads, low-cost meals, no dining out, no movies or clubs, no shopping for clothes.

Roberta felt really good about herself. The first two days, she handled herself well. She'd taken $100 out of the bank and she still had $65 left in her wallet—and another $230 in her account. But the third day? Roberta was web-surfing and came across a brand-new "miracle" cream. It was supposed to get rid of dark cycles under the eyes, wrinkles, redness; it guaranteed glowing skin. But it was $225 a jar. Roberta knew she didn't have the money, and she quickly escaped to another site. But the cream gnawed at her. She'd think about it when she brushed her teeth and when she was driving to work. Finally, Roberta couldn't stand it anymore; she had to buy the cream. She charged it, using her debit card, which soon left her with a minus balance in her account.

During the next week, the bank fees that Roberta was charged when checks were returned more than equaled the cost of the cream! Why did she do it? By the time the cream came, Roberta was so anxious that she was tempted to return it—but she didn't.

She liked the way it looked on her skin. The cream felt great, yes, but now she was broke. And very anxious about money.

Call it generalized anxiety disorder. Call it separation anxiety. Call it delusional behavior. Call it denial. Call it agoraphobic, any sort of phobic. Whatever you call it, the underlying symptoms are exuberance and anxiety, and if they are later followed by a downswing, they may signal bipolar II.

Although substance abuse and bipolar have been researched, studied, and analyzed in countless articles, bipolar combined with anxiety has not—despite the fact that anxiety disorders and bipolar disease are more prevalent than substance abuse.[1] Over half the bipolar patients in one study (55.8 percent) had at least one co-existing anxiety disorder; almost one-third of the patients (31.8 percent) had more than one.[2] Panic disorder is the most common form of anxiety, appearing both in hypomaniac cycles and in people caught in a depressed and manic cycle."[3] Generalized anxiety disorder (GAD) is the most common form of anxiety found in bipolar disorder as a whole.[4]

The Four Types of Manic Anxiety

You know it when you're feeling anxious, that lip-biting, heart-dropping, leg-shaking fear before a test, a presentation, or an interview. But "normal" folk ease back to their calm state once the anxiety-producing situation is over. People with bipolar II are not so lucky. When one stressor disappears, another takes its place. The anxiety stays. It's only the situations that change.

Because anxiety is so prevalent with bipolar disorder (as well as with depression) and is a part of a bipolar II "high," we need to explore it. This section will detail the different types of common anxiety diagnoses to see whether one fits you. Although

• MIXED UP

Although it sounds like a contradiction of terms, people can have both mania and depression at the same time. This "mixed state" is characterized by anxiety and hostility, anxiety and moodiness, anxiety and hopelessness, aggressiveness and low self-esteem, racing thoughts and restlessness. People with bipolar II are more susceptible to mixed states than those with bipolar I or major depression. However, they are less prone to "rapid cycling," in which mania becomes depression, and vice versa, within the course of a week, a day, or even the same hour. People with bipolar II tend to stay depressed for longer periods of time.

How to keep up? Eventually, as I did, you become very sensitive to your body and its signals and adjust your medication accordingly. (If you experience shifts in your moods while on medication, make sure you speak to your psychiatrist—who should be aware of your anxiety and your mood shifts.)

each anxiety disorder has its own category in the DSM-IV-TR, if yours is a component of bipolar II—that is, if it is not depression or a "stand-alone" anxiety disorder—treatment will usually be the same for all of them. Let's look at four "worrying kinds," or types, of anxiety that are commonly seen with bipolar disease.

"Worrying Kind" 1: Generalized Anxiety Disorder (GAD)

This was me—anxious about anything and everything. The doctors I'd been seeing chalked my symptoms up to a female constitution and gave me antianxiety medication. The meds they prescribed calmed me for a few hours, but I became addicted and was taking one, two, or even three Ativans a day. (I was also smoking about three packs of cigarettes at the time.) And since I was only being treated for part of my disorder, ultimately nothing was effective—until I got the right diagnosis.

According to a 2004 paper published in the *Journal of Clinical Psychiatry*, 31.2 percent of people with bipolar disorder suffer from GAD.[5]

FIGURE 3-1. Signs of GAD[6]

- An inability to "shake off" worries and concerns in all facets of your life
- An inability to stop worrying about concerns you know intellectually are minor or imagined
- Insomnia
- An inability to relax
- Fatigue and muscle aches
- Headaches
- Irritability
- Trembling and twitching, your whole body affected
- Sweating
- Difficulty swallowing

"Worrying Kind" 2: Panic Disorder

Jane was in a friend's living room, along with several other friends. It was a small gathering; they were making small talk and sipping cocktails while their hostess was in the kitchen. Jane knew only one of the other people, but she was already chatting with the person sharing the couch, a glass of wine in hand. Jane was a bit nervous; she hadn't slept much the night before and there were a lot of pressures at work. But she assumed she was handling herself just fine.

Then, a few minutes after she'd sipped her wine, she felt dizzy. She couldn't breathe. Her mouth went dry and her heart was pounding. She jumped up. "Someone spiked my drink!" she shouted.

In reality, no one had done any such thing, and Jane was mortified. Her symptoms, albeit frightening, showed all the characteristics of panic disorder. According to a 2004 paper in the *Journal of Clinical Psychiatry*, 26.8 percent of people with bipolar disorder suffer from panic disorder.[7]

FIGURE 3-2. Signs of Panic Disorder[8]

- Feelings of terror that strike suddenly with no warning
- Recurrent feelings of terror
- Pounding, racing heart
- Feeling light-headed, dizzy, and/or weak
- Feeling as if you are going to faint
- Breaking out in a sweat
- Tingling, numb hands
- Feeling chilled or flushed
- Nausea
- Symptoms lasting approximately 10 minutes

"Worrying Kind" 3: Obsessive-Compulsive Disorder (OCD)

OCD conjures up a variety of clichés: stacks of newspapers and debris literally taking over an apartment, washing hands over and over, compulsively counting, straightening rows and picture frames: The television character Monk without his nurse. People with OCD are usually less concerned with themselves than with those they love. "What if . . ." is their mantra, and they are unable to stop the compulsive behavior that somewhat relieves their obsessive worrying about their family, their friends, the world.

In the minds of people with OCD, the ritualistic behavior can stop a terrible thing from happening—even though they intellectually know that's not the way things work. But the "power" from the compulsive behavior lasts only until another thought pops into their heads. Ultimately, the ritual to assuage the anxiety controls them. For example, Lisa, a member of an OCD support group, believed that whenever she went past an empty lot, her family house would catch fire and everyone would be burned. In order to stop this horror from happening, she had to walk back and forth past the lot five times before moving on. If she was in a car? She'd literally have to go around the block five times. A number of famous people, such as Winston Churchill, Frances Ford Coppola, J. P. Morgan, Alvin Ailley, and Jose Conseco, have suffered from OCD.[9]

FIGURE 3-3. Signs of OCD[10]

- Persistent, unwelcome thoughts or images
- Continuous rumination
- An urgent need to perform a ritual (behavior)
- Obsession with objects, such as germs and dirt, or with more ambiguous subjects, such as health, cleanliness, and safety
- A feeling of doubt that makes you feel very anxious
- A need to check things over and over again
- An overriding anxiety that is eased temporarily by performing a ritual

"Worrying Kind" 4: Social Anxiety Disorder

Social anxiety disorder, or social phobia, is one of the most common forms of anxiety—in people with or without bipolar disorder. Its basic definition is the acute anxiety and self-consciousness felt in everyday situations; it's the "butterflies in the stomach" taken to warp speed, where a person is literally unable to perform, go to school, or speak. According to one study, 15 percent of people suffer from social phobia before giving a speech. Participating in a meeting came in second, with 14 percent, followed by walking into a room where others are already seated, 13 percent.[11] Other social phobias include fear of eating or drinking in public or of going to school. According to the same 2004 paper published in the *Journal of Clinical Psychiatry*, 17.4 percent of people with bipolar disorder suffer from social anxiety disorder.[12]

FIGURE 3-4. Signs of Social Anxiety Disorder[13]

- Persistent, overwhelming, and acute fear of being watched and judged by others
- Persistent, chronic fear of being embarrassed or humiliated by one's own actions
- Fear continues even after the situation has passed
- Fear is so intense that it interferes with work, school, and other activities
- Blushing, sweating, trembling, and an inability to talk when confronted with a situation that causes fear

"Anxiety is nearly always part of bipolar disorder," says Dr. Andrea Fagiolini, M.D., psychiatrist and medical director of the Bipolar Center at the University of Pittsburgh School of Medicine. As reported by Jeanie Lerche Davis in an interview with WebMD, he continues: "Not only is it difficult to distingush between anxiety and mania, it is sometimes impossible."[14]

But whether full-blown anxiety or mania, the "high" goes away eventually . . . and in its place? Depression—mania's polar opposite and the emotional state we'll be discussing next.

4

Swing Low the Bipolar II Way
Depression

The madness of depression is the antithesis of violence. It is a storm indeed, but a storm of murk.

—WILLIAM STYRON

LIKE THE TWIN masks of comedy and drama, hot and cold, heads or tails, bipolar II has its very un-hypomanic side. Whether you plunge into depression from a hypomanic state or from a state of manic anxiety, if you have bipolar II, depression is going to hit sooner or later. And, with bipolar II, it will hang around much longer than the flip side.

Many people who have this condition experience depressive episodes that usually last longer than two weeks—and sometimes last two years or more. In fact, it's the long-term depression that has most people with bipolar II contacting a doctor for the first time—which is why bipolar II is so often misdiagnosed as clinical depression.[1]

And just to mix up the brew, bipolar II exhibits atypical signs of depression. In other words, some of the depressive symptoms might not look like unipolar depression at all.

Craig's Story

Take Craig, for example. When Craig got depressed, the onset was never gradual. His depressive episodes weren't slow erosions of his psyche. Instead, he'd be extra-confident and wired one day, and then—boom—he'd start to feel bad. But because his demeanor changed so abruptly, those around him attributed it to overwork and the stress of a new job. No one suspected he was depressed, because he pretended he was fine and "faked it" very well. Sure, he drank a lot, but everyone did. There was nothing like a few beers after work to unwind. But for Craig, the alcohol helped numb his pain—to an extent.

Craig had gotten a plum job right out of architecture school: he was hired as an assistant to a famous architect. At first he was ecstatic. He'd come to work brimming with enthusiasm and energy; he was ready to take on the world (or at least Chicago, where the firm was based). But even though his enthusiasm never waned, he started to feel anxious. While passing people in conversation in the hall, he wondered if they were talking about him; when his boss didn't thank him for completing a task, he wondered if he was getting fired. These feelings were embarrassing and Craig tried to ignore them. Guys didn't worry about stuff like that, or at least they didn't talk about it.

One day, Craig woke up feeling horrible. He was exhausted despite having slept eight hours; he had no energy, and all of a sudden, he hated his job. He hated being anxious, he hated worrying, he hated working all hours, and most of all, he hated himself. Who was he trying to kid? He wasn't architect material! His self-esteem was nonexistent; he felt hopeless and helpless, and he couldn't understand it. Just last night, over cocktails, one of his co-workers had told him the work was he was doing great!

But the anxiety that had been his companion for several weeks had run its course. Craig's unrelenting, full throttle anxiety went into slow motion. He'd start to worry and then go to sleep. He'd wake up, start to worry, and go back to sleep. He was exhausted; he had a pounding headache; his muscles ached as if he'd just run ten miles. He called in sick—day after day. At first, everyone sent "get well soon" wishes, but when three days turned into five, and five into ten, it became unacceptable. His boss wanted him to go to the doctor. Craig told him he would, but once he hung up the phone, he just went back to sleep. He didn't want to lose his job, but another part of him didn't care. He was afraid he had an illness, but another part of him wanted him to stay sick. He was frozen, unable to do anything but eat and sleep. After several warnings about his absenteeism, the firm finally had no choice but to fire him.

The result? Craig could finally sleep in peace. He'd get dressed in some sweats in the morning and pick up food at the deli down the street: Twinkies, grilled cheese sandwiches, peanut butter, ice cream, chips, crackers, and chocolate bars. He began gaining weight from this diet and his inactivity. He also stopped trying to pretend. He canceled dates, and even though he started to read the want ads each morning, by mid-afternoon he had crawled into bed.

Craig's friends began to worry. His behavior could no longer be attributed to getting fired. It was time to "snap out of it" and get on with his life. They thought maybe he was lazy and self-indulgent. It couldn't be depression. After all, Craig slept a lot, and wasn't insomnia one of the telltale symptoms of depression? And he wasn't losing weight—another red flag for depression. If anything, he was getting fat. And there was no "spiraling down," slowly becoming more and more depressed. Could Craig have become depressed practically overnight?

Craig's girlfriend finally got him to see a psychiatrist, who was able to make a diagnosis almost immediately: major depression. She recommended antidepressants and talk therapy. All the meds did, however, was make Craig feel more hyper; he still hated himself. And he didn't get better.

But he did get lucky. The second psychiatrist he started to see made the correct diagnosis. Although the average amount of time it takes a patient to get a correct diagnosis of bipolar II is ten years, it took Craig only four.

What Is Bipolar II Depression?

Just as we know when we are anxious, we also know when we're feeling depressed. We might deny it, we might avoid getting help, but that hopeless and helpless feeling doesn't go away. If anything, it gets worse over time.

In major depression, or unipolar depression, a person's moods don't switch like a pendulum, mania to depression, depression to mania. A person stays depressed, and any anxiety she experiences is the result of that depression: her isolation, her feelings of inadequacy, her ruminations over events just past or in the future. Determining whether your depression is unipolar or bipolar takes expertise on a physician's part, a battery of tests, and self-knowledge. Have you gone through a particularly stressful time for over six months, finding yourself feeling more and more hopeless? Have you experienced a loss that, months later, still felt as if it had just occurred?

If the depression is something you've never experienced before and it's been hanging around for more than a month, you could very well have bipolar II. In fact, your bipolar hypomania can skip mania and, instead, plunge you into a major depression—often before you've had a chance to "enjoy" your hypomanic state. (See Figure 4-1 for easy reference to the symptoms of depression in bipolar II; you can also find this list in Chapter 1, Figure 1-2.)

FIGURE 4-1. In Depressive Cycle [2]

Early and usually abrupt onset, recurrent and lasting 3 to 6 months:

Hypersomnia (sleeping too much)
Weight gain
Self-pity
Somatization (the manic cycle's anxiety turned into physical problems)
Depressive feelings that are worse in the evening
Unrelenting jealousy
Suspicion and paranoia
Difficult, demanding behavior
Extreme sensitivity to rejection
Narcissistic misinterpretation of people's actions and words (called ideas of reference)
Slowing down of motor skills (psychomotor retardation)
Excessive feelings of guilt
Depersonalization (losing one's self-identity and sense of reality)
Withdrawal and isolation
Derealization (alterations in perception in which familiar things "feel strange")
Suicidal ideation (thoughts)

• "SINGLE-CYCLE" DEPRESSION

Unipolar depression, unlike bipolar, does not have a manic component. People with clinical depression may exhibit either atypical or more traditional signs and symptoms of depression. Without proper treatment, the depressed individual can spiral further and further down until suicide is attempted.

The depressive symptoms seen in bipolar II are usually what clinicians call atypical depression—a term coined in the 1950s to describe a number of patients in a London hospital who did not respond to either electroshock therapy or the conventional antidepressants of the day.[3]

Atypical depression (AD) is actually a misnomer. Ironically, what was considered atypical in the mid-twentieth century is very typical today. It is seen in all clinical settings—from physician offices to hospitals—and as many as one-third of those diagnosed with depression have characteristics of the atypical kind.[4] A 1998 National Comorbidity Survey, which gathered information on patients ranging from young adults to those in midlife, found that has many as 40 percent of people who were depressed showed atypical symptoms.[5] But even a diagnosis of AD isn't enough for those of us with bipolar II. In fact, antidepressants may "push" people with bipolar disorder into a manic state.

In addition to an atypical depression, a person with bipolar can also have an "atypical" bipolar: *cyclothymia*. Although it might sound like a bad made-for-television sci-fi movie, cyclothymia is simply a condition in which a person has chronic mood swings for two years or more, but whose hypomanic and depressive symptoms do not become mania or major depression. Think of it as the low-fat version of bipolar II.

• UP AND DOWN, DOWN AND UP

Another characteristic of bipolar II depression is rapid cycling, which is characterized by four or more episodes of depression, mania, mixed states, or hypomania within a twelve-month period, each one lasting more than two months.[6]

People with bipolar II are 15 percent more likely to be rapid cyclers than their bipolar I counterparts.[7] Because atypical depressions are also more receptive to outside events, people with bipolar usually swing quickly from AD to a hypomanic (or manic) state if something positive happens in their lives.

Depression in bipolar II is insidious because it is so frequently misdiagnosed. In one epidemiological study, the *first* 600 respondents to a mental health questionnaire were misdiagnosed. Ultimately, the study suggested that 69 percent of people with bipolar disorder are initially misdiagnosed.[8] And the most common misdiagnosis? You guessed it. Depression. In another study, 72 percent people with bopolar disorder were misdiagnosed with unipolar (major) depression.[9]

What makes this misdiagnosis worse is the fact that the depressive cycle is three times more prevalent than its manic counterpart.[10] And without the proper diagnosis, people with bipolar will have less positive quality of life. They are more likely to have lower income, lower job status, and poorer relationships than their healthier counterparts.[11]

There's more to bipolar disorder than the highs and the lows. There's the chemistry involved, the temperament you were born with, and genetics—all of which we'll explore in the next section, which addresses the question "Why do I have bipolar II?"

PART TWO

Why Do I Have Bipolar II?

5

The Bipolar Brain

The brain is wider than the sky.
—EMILY DICKINSON

THERE'S AN EXPRESSION used when a person has a stroke and every minute counts: "Time is brain." For those of us with a mental disorder, I would change it to "*Timing* is brain."

There is no physical collapse, no black or white, no immediate life and death struggle with mental disorders. It's the way the chemicals in your brain interact, the way your brain, your blood, your genes, and even your instincts come together at birth and during your life experiences that makes you who you are today—and these factors also contribute to your having bipolar II. You may be predisposed to the condition via the genes you inherited from your parents and the way your chemistry is set up, but it takes the way you react to a situation—some kind of stress—to ignite it. In other words, timing.

An esteemed child psychiatrist once told me that he has seen healthy teenagers raised by the most horrendous of parents, and he has seen children afflicted with depression or bipolar disorder raised by parents who'd win a "Best Parent" award. In short, in many cases, the reason why you and not someone else has bipolar disorder is the "luck of the draw."[1] Timing is everything.

But "how" is as important as "why." In order to truly understand what physically occurs in the brain to create mental disorders, you first have to understand the way the brain works.

A Journey through the Brain

If you've graduated from high school, you probably have had to dissect a frog. (I can still remember, with horror, the dead, flayed frog on its metal slab, the odor of formaldehyde so strong it "drowned out" even the sounds of my classmates in biology lab.) It's difficult to believe, but that minute ball, that peanut of a brain you exposed in the frog, is much like our own—that, in fact, the brain that tells our heart to pump blood, our lungs to breathe in and out, our glands to produce more hormones in the face of danger is functionally the same as a frog's.

The only thing separating our brain from those of lesser animals is a more sophisticated "emotional-memory-thinking axis" located in the area near and in the cerebral cortex: here our thinking, analyzing, discovering, hoping, and fears arise.

Very quickly, then, let's travel through the parts of the brain that ultimately lead to the complex, maze-like, electrically charged, and chemically fueled cerebral cortex that makes us who we are. (For a visual counterpoint to these descriptions, refer to Figure 5-1.)

The Beginning: The Peripheral Nervous System and Brainstem

The peripheral nervous system, the network of nerve passageways that twist and turn through every part of our body, is ex-

Figure 5-1. A Cross Section of the Brain

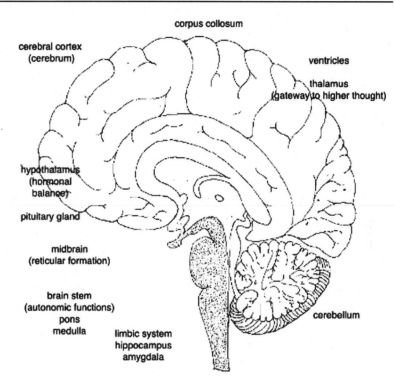

Drawing by Frances Pelzman Liscio

actly that: it is peripheral and secondary, with all of its roads, laden with stimuli and responses, leading to the spinal cord. From here on out, the central nervous system (CNS), consisting of the spinal cord and the brain, takes over.

Within the bony structure of our spine, nerves, laden with messages, shoot up and down like one of those tubes at a drive-in bank. The juncture where the thick nerve fibers of the spinal cord meet the brain is called the brainstem, home to all the automatic functions we share with the frog: breathing, swallowing, regulating blood pressure, and maintaining body temperature. A little farther up the road, but still considered a part of the brainstem, is the midbrain, where other automatic responses, such as eye muscle movement, reflexes, and alertness, are supervised.[2]

An area of the brainstem called the raphe nucleus is where serotonin, a neurotransmitter closely associated with bipolar disorder and depression, is created and then dispersed to different parts of the brain. Studies show that there is 40 percent less of a particular genetic marker (the 1a receptor) in the neurons responsible for serotonin in people with bipolar disorder.[3]

• STOP AND SMELL . . .

The brainstem controls our every sense except sight and smell. These two go directly to higher parts of the brain without stopping, which explains why these senses are always felt more acutely—why, for example, a certain scent can transport you in an instant to the backseat of your first car or a flash of color in a scarf can poignantly evoke the image of your deceased mother.[4]

The entire brainstem looks very much like a reptile's complete brain—indeed, it is sometimes called the reptilian brain. The next time you wonder why a frog (a live one) can't add two plus two, you'll know it's because its brain stops here.

Getting Closer: The Cerebellum

No, the cerebellum is not the era Scarlett O'Hara lived in. It is Latin for "little brain" and it's attached to the back of the brainstem. This "little brain" is not that small when you consider that it coordinates all our movements, our every step, our every stance; it even coordinates the muscles that help us speak. It also stores some of our simple, ingrained memories—from singing the words to "Happy Birthday" to saying thank you when someone hands you a gift. So far, a person with bipolar II has the same wiring as someone who doesn't. We really aren't that different after all.

Almost There: The Thalamus and Hypothalamus

Above the brainstem and in front of the cerebellum are the highly efficient thalamus and hypothalamus—the gateways to our thoughts, emotions, and, separating the wheat from the chaff, our mental health.

Every bit of information, and every message from the insignificant to the sublime, goes through the thalamus—a "Google" of sorts that does a preliminary search before determining what part of the brain gets what message. For example, say you see a great dress in a Macy's window. The thalamus directs the image of that dress to go to your memory storage banks located in the higher areas of the brain. At the same time, your emotions are heightened as you think about how you'll look at the party wearing that dress. (For a person with bipolar II, that emotion may be awash with anxiety.) The cost of the dress is also a matter for the higher parts of your brain to access—and one that the thalamus gives short shrift in a manic state. Your thalamus is continually directing traffic, bouncing these thoughts (or messages) about the dress to different parts of the higher brain, making sure that all components of The Dress are covered—from fit, color, and excitement, to checkbook balance, credit card limit, and, if you're in the early throes of hypomania, extreme bliss.

Right below the thalamus is the hypothalamus, the brain's hormonal control tower. Although no bigger than the size of a pea, it's a dynamo of function, regulating our eating patterns, our sleeping and waking cycles, our sex drive, and, crucially for people with any mental disorder, our pituitary gland. The pituitary is the king, queen, and royal staff of hormonal (chemical) secretion, the mighty regulator of the hormones that feed our basic and higher functions. In other words, without the help of the hypothalamus, you won't be able to get much further evolved than the frog.[5]

A close neighbor to the thalamus is the ventral striatum, a part of the brain that helps process rewards. Studies show overactivity in this corner of the brain (and 30 percent less gray matter) in people with bipolar disorder. The result? Poor judgment—an inability to understand that overspending or promiscuity can adversely affect their lives.[6]

• IN CASE YOU ARE ON *JEOPARDY* AND THE CATEGORY IS "THE BRAIN"

- Your whole brain weighs about three pounds and is about the size of a bag of sugar.
- Your skin weighs twice as much as your brain.
- There are over 100 billion nerve cells in the basic brain—which is about 165 times the population of Earth.
- The brain is 75 percent water.
- By the time you are seven years old, your brain is almost adult in weight and size.
- All babies start out with a female-like brain. A male's brain develops different circuitry when the male hormone, testosterone, is pumped up to the brain, usually after eight weeks of life.
- It takes only eight to ten seconds for a brain deprived of its blood supply to become unconscious.[7]

Bipolar II Brain Destinations

Although the thalamus, hypothalamus, and other areas of the middle brain come into play in mental illness, most aspects of brain dysfunction occur in the next few segments, where higher brain functions, such as logic, emotion, and conceptualizing take place.

The Emotional Limbic System

Stimulate a section of a cat's hypothalamus and you'll see an un-provoked hissing and frenzied attack. Stimulate a different section and suddenly you'll have a purring kitty that wants to sit on your lap. But these behaviors have taken place in a vacuum. In neither case has the cat been provoked; it isn't angry—nor is it necessarily loving. Yes, the cat had most definitely "acted out" a behavioral response, but without any underlying emotion.

That's where the limbic system comes in. This network of nerve cells endows us with the capacity to feel; it supplies the emotional tone of our actions. It adds the depth missing from the cat's "sham" rage and from its empty purr. Thanks to the limbic system, we can feel true anger, sadness, joy, and elation. In the case of someone with bipolar disorder, the limbic system presents over-the-top versions of these same emotions.

Because it's nestled right below the higher-functioning cerebral parts of the brain, the limbic system ensures that emotions reach our conscious thoughts—and that our thoughts affect our emotions. Both the limbic system and the higher-functioning parts of the brain actively influence one another. A chemical imbalance can provoke the wrong triggers and/or create an inappropriate response to an event or situation. For example, an imbalanced limbic system can make us passively shrug off the time we were stood up (or, conversely, imprint the memory with terror). It can also make us feel depressed even when we are among a group of supportive friends.[8]

The Memorable Hippocampus and Amygdala

They might sound like characters from the cast of *Cats,* but in reality, the hippocampus and the amygdala are responsible for much of what we remember.

The hippocampus looks like a seahorse and is conveniently located in the front of your brain to connect directly to your senses, your memories—and your limbic system.

The hippocampus can pick up, say, the vision of a bright summer day, along with its flowery scent wafting through a breeze, and connect this vision with a memory of a similar summer day when you were a kid, a memory it's been storing for maybe twenty years! Thanks to this capacity, the hippocampus can spur the limbic system into action, evoking the emotion of nostalgia. And this emotion, in turn, helps trigger the thinking areas of the brain, which will open the floodgates on the past and and all the thoughts, promises, and long-ago dreams that past implies.

This rush of memory and its emotional images are enhanced by the amygdala, which sits right in the middle of the limbic system. The amygdala also helps people recognize facial expressions and tones of voice—which are often incorrectly interpreted in people with bipolar disorder. Chemical imbalances in the brain may also affect the amygdala's function, so that, for example, a person with bipolar II may not "read" another person accurately. In fact, studies have shown that people with bipolar disorder may actually see a negative expression when the other person is merely being neutral. In other words, people with bipolar II perceive a neutral expression as disapproving. (My therapist calls it being an anti-psychic.) The amygdala in people with bipolar disorder may also remain active long after the annoyed boss or "I told you so" friend has left the building—which means you may continue to feel fearful, angry, or sad much longer than is appropriate.

The subiculum, another area of the hippocampus, uses stored memory to help people recognize situations that may be dangerous or rewarding—and it, too, is "skewed" in people with bipolar disorder. There are fewer connections to the subiculum, and this means that you can't always tell whether a situation is safe.[9] Given the anxiety I've lived with for over forty years, I'd say my subiculum is most likely scrubbed clean.

The Civilized Cerebral Cortex

The mighty cerebral cortex is the quintessential area of the brain that makes us who we are and how we function in the outside world. It's the part of the brain where we organize and abstract, communicate and appreciate, create, perceive, remember, and analyze—all those activities of thought and problem solving that we call "executive function." In other words, it's the place where we think.

But, for all its deep thoughts, the cerebral cortex is physically very superficial. It is actually a thin blanket made of nerves, an eighth-of-an-inch-thick layer of billions and billions of cells. Underneath it, warm and snug, is the bulk of the brain, the chunky white matter that scientists call the cerebrum. The more you know, the more your brain grows. But rather than our heads coming to resemble the enormous brow of an imagined alien from space, swollen smooth with learning, our life experiences and lessons increase only the surface of our brain. The growing cerebral cortex folds and rolls over the cerebrum, giving our brains their classic wrinkled, crinkled appearance.

Gray, drab, and slender, the cerebral cortex looks completely uninspiring. But don't be fooled—it holds what makes us human, what makes us individuals, and what makes us *ourselves*. It's also where messages can become distorted, unreal, and misunderstood—where mental illness may take hold and, combined with the limbic system's emotions, may hang on for dear life.[10]

• LOBE-TROTTING

Like a patchwork quilt, the cerebral cortex blanket is also divided into segments and halves. In your mind's eye, draw a magic marker down the middle, dividing the brain in half. Each of these halves, called hemispheres, is a mirror image of the other, with different functioning. The left hemisphere is associated with logic, problem solving, and language; the right hemisphere is associated with your visual memories and your ability to make art, play music, or dance.

But the brain doesn't stop here. Each hemisphere is also divided into four segments called lobes. The right hemisphere of the brain has four right lobes and the left has (you guessed it) four left lobes. Each lobe has specific functions. The frontal lobes house our executive functions; the occipital lobes interpret our sight; the temporal lobes store much of our memory; and the parietal lobes help bring letters together as words—and turn words into thoughts. Figure 5-2 illustrates the different lobes and shows how they are divided in the brain. By isolating each section, researchers are able to pinpoint more clearly where a chemical malfunction is taking place.

The Crux of the Matter: Communication

All this brain anatomy has been leading up to this: the way messages (or stimuli) from the outside are deciphered in the brain and travel back to the outside (response). It is here—as messages move up to your midbrain, down to your heart, up to your limbic system, across your temporal lobe, back and forth in the cerebral cortex, down your spinal cord, through your thalamus, and past your hippocampus—that the roots of bipolar II can take hold. The pathways these messages take across your brain determine, just as decisively as life events that occur outside your body, whether or not you'll feel happy, whether or not your behavior is unacceptable, whether or not you are so depressed you can barely function.

Figure 5-2. The Lobes of the Brain

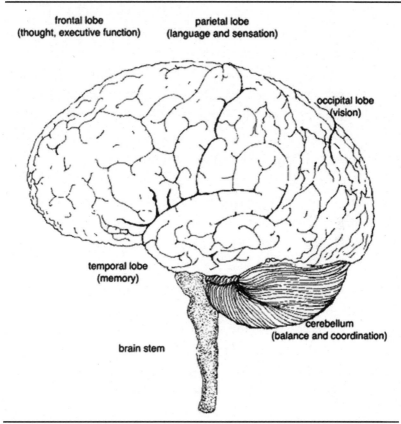

frontal lobe
(thought, executive function)

parietal lobe
(language and sensation)

occipital lobe
(vision)

temporal lobe
(memory)

cerebellum
(balance and coordination)

brain stem

Drawing by Frances Pelzman Liscio

Using a very simplified stimulus-response pair (*dripping wet—grab a towel*), here's how one particular message gets past the frog and into the essence of who we are. As you stand fresh from your shower, the water dripping down your back, you feel wet. The stimulus *wet* bounces back and forth from the brainstem (where your temperature may drop and your skin develop goose bumps) up to your limbic system (where you'll feel miserable and uncomfortable) to your frontal lobe (where you think

you'll catch a cold unless—aha!—you dry off). The response—
dry off—will bounce from your optical lobe (where you'll perceive the towel on the rack) to your hypothalamus (where a
request for adrenaline keeps you on your toes), from your temporal lobe (where you'll remember how good a dry towel feels)
back to your frontal lobe (where you'll demand the #(*$! towel
already). And it has to do all this while millions of other messages—from breathing to scratching an itch, from thinking
about dinner to remembering a deadline at work, from feeling
anxious about that deadline to actually sitting down and doing
the work—are *also* traveling the same brain highway. All the
time, an infinite number of commands are being shouted, information is being stored, perceptions are being understood, emotions are being felt, and all are being perfectly relayed in your
brain in less than a second, every hour of the day and even as
you sleep.

There's a reason why computers and fiber optics are often used
to describe the brain. Just as we send an e-mail through cyber-
space via cable, satellite, or cell phone, the brain and the entire
nervous system have a network of signals and wires that connect
every part of that system to other parts. These wires are nerve
cells called neurons. They carry messages like *dripping wet—grab
a towel* via both electrical impulses and chemical conductors.
Here's how:

An electrical impulse, carrying, say, the message *icy cold,* will
travel along a neuron's cell body until it gets to the edge of the
cell, its *axon.* There, in front of the axon, is a small space in
the road called a *synapse.* Think of it as a river without a bridge.
The electrical impulse cannot cross the "river." In order to get
across the synapse to the next neuron and continue carrying its
message, the impulse must change from an electrical "car" into a

chemical "boat," or, in clinical terms, into a *neurotransmitter.* Once across the synapse, the message converts back into electricity, and the entire electrochemical process repeats at the next neuron's edge. (See Figure 5-3 for a magnified look at a neuron and Figure 5-4 for a magnified view of a neurotransmitter and synapse.)

It is at this synapse, where electric current meets chemical neurotransmitter, that mental disorders ignite.

Figure 5-3. A Cross Section of a Neuron

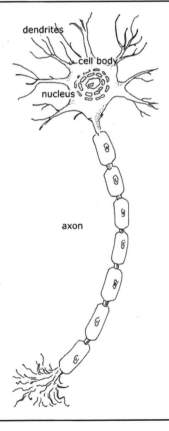

Drawing by Frances Pelzman Liscio

Figure 5-4. A Magnified View of the Relationship between Neurotransmitter and Synapse

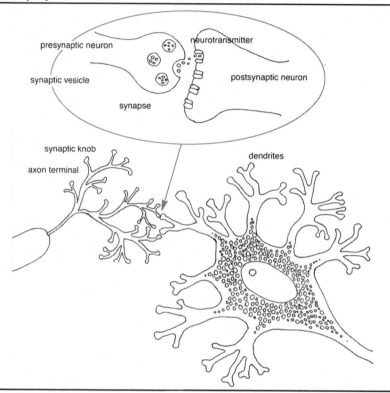

Drawing by Frances Pelzman Liscio

When Good Chemicals Go Bad

As difficult as it is to envision the frog's brain as part of your own physiology, it's watching an episode of *Teletubbies* compared to envisioning how a microscopically small trace of a chemical in the brain can create despair, anxiety, suicidal thoughts, or mania.

But just as a strand of amino acid proteins called DNA dictates the color of our eyes, our ability to play piano, and our predilection toward math, the amount and/or reaction of specific chemicals in the brain can make the difference between having bipolar II and not having this disorder.

Basically, those lines of communication from neuron to neuron stay active only as long as the chemicals, the neurotransmitters, in the synaptic bridge respond. Some neurotransmitters are "excitatory"; they're meant to jazz up your wiring (get a dry towel—pronto!). Others are "inhibitory"; they're meant to subdue (no rushing naked to a nearby Bed & Bath!). If an electromechanical message gets to the edge of a neuron but there's no chemical receptor "boat" to guide it across to the next neuron, that message will die. Similarly, if a receptor gets its signals crossed so that the message carried forth is misread, or if there's already a full neurotransmitter "boat" with no room for one more, the message will be corrupted, be changed, or die. And once that happens, the message will falter, a chemical imbalance will occur, and the message may forever be tinged with mental disorder—unless specific medications or lifestyle activities change its course.

• 1,000+PIECES

Each neurotransmitter will respond only to one specific neuron. Like pieces of a jigsaw puzzle, there has to be an exact match for a message to fly across the synapse to the next neuron. Without the right electrical "password," a neurotransmitter will lie silent or be mistakenly activated.

That's not always a bad thing. Not every neurotransmitter sitting in a synapse *should* have a match. In fact, many neurotransmitters need to be silent in order for the correct message to get through. The newest research on brain injury, whether from a stroke or an accident, shows that when the trauma occurs, a cascade of excited neurotransmitters race to the injury site; neurotransmitters that would normally be silent, still, and quiet are activated. The result? More damage to the brain.[10]

C'est Moi Mon Amie

In mood disorders like bipolar II, the neurotransmitters (read: chemicals) are out of whack, with some chemicals responding more and other chemicals responding less. The imbalanced neurotransmitters most frequently found in mood disorders are monoamines, so classified because they all have an amino acid composition in common. A study published in the *American Journal of Psychiatry* found that people with bipolar disorder had 30 percent more monoamines than those who did not have the disorder.[11] Monoamines affect mood, ability to experience reward and pleasure, concentration, stress regulation, and ability to pay attention.

The three monoamines most associated with bipolar disorder are

Serotonin, involved in the regulation of sleep, mood, memory, and temperature regulation. It has also been found to influence appetite, migraine headaches, and anxiety. Studies have found that a serotonin imbalance is behind overeating; simple carbohydrates increase activity levels and make you feel better.

Norepinephrine, affecting your ability to focus and pay attention. An imbalance of norepinpephrine may also cause depression.

Dopamine, affecting emotion, movement, and perception.

Because of recent advances in scientific research into brain chemistry, medicine today can be more effective. Various types of antidepressants and anticonvulsants affect the activity of monoamines and, depending on your particular brain structure, will work to recreate chemical balance in the brain. (See Chapter 9 for details on pharmaceutical medications for bipolar II.)

• CHEMICALLY SPEAKING

Monoamines aren't the only neurotransmitters in the house. Here are some other chemicals associated with bipolar disease:

Glutamate is both an amino acid (a building block of DNA) and a neurotransmitter. It moves fast when activated, affecting memory and the way we learn.

GABA, or gamma-aminobutyric acid for short, controls inhibition. Not enough in your system will produce mania; drugs that increase GABA are often used to treat mania. (But the reduction of mania may also be a result of the sedative effect of the drugs.)

Acetylcholine has the distinction of being the first neurotransmitter to have been discovered (in the 1920s). It affects memory and learning and is also linked to Alzheimer's disease.

Chemical Theories at Large

Do frogs have neurotransmitters? Yes. Do they have excitatory and inhibitory neurotransmitters? Yes. Can their neurotransmitters be corrupted or changed? Yes. And studies show that their environment—a dried-up swamp, a lake filled with insects—plays a role in those changing neurotransmitters.[12] But that's as far as it goes. A frog doesn't realize that it's going to die for a high school biology class; it isn't even aware that it exists.

We humans, on the other hand, are rich in neurotransmitters that spark or quiet past and present thoughts, that draw conclusions, that predict the future and keep dreams alive. And we are learning more and more about how our neurotransmitters "speak" to each other every day—and how that language affects not only who we are but also why some of us have mental disorders. A sampling:

DARPP-32 and Dopamine

In 2000, Nobel Prize winners Erick Kandel, M.D., and Arvid Carlsson, Ph.D., discovered a molecule, dubbed DARPP-32, that influences dopamine production—a chemical central to our feeling pleasure.[13] In 2003, the National Institutes of Mental Health went a step further with this discovery. They found that it's not the neurotransmitter at the synaptic bridge that affects our behavior, but the configuration of the neuron itself—and how it is affected by DARPP-32—that influences the way we process information. In other words, there is no good or bad gene, no "crazy" or "normal" gene; there are only different levels of processing. And dopamine, long thought an significant cousin to serotonin and norepinephrine, was found possibly to be more important in defining our moods.[14] By balancing our serotonin levels, for example, antidepressants are also making us more responsive to DARPP-32 and, subsequently, to dopamine. And the more dopamine in our brains, the better we feel.

Spindle Cells

Off-color jokes about cigars notwithstanding, spindle neuron cells, shaped like microscopic cigars, are harbingers of moral consciousness. Although not present at birth, by the time you are two or three, they are in place in the frontal cortex and are activated during risky or provocative situations (just about when guilt and embarrassment start to rear their sometimes ugly heads). As you develop more moral judgment, more spindle cells appear. The greater your capacity to understand complex emotions, the more spindle cells you have.[15] They affect the ability to experience adult emotions and the capability to solve problems.

The VMpo and the Insula

It might sound like a Greek tragedy, but in reality, it's what enables you to experience the emotional impact of the play. The VMpo, or posterior ventromedial nucleus, lies just in back of the thalamus. An enormous part of the brain in humans, the VMpo collects information that has come up from other areas of the brain—from the basics, such as keeping body temperature stable, to the more complex, such as the layers of emotion we are experiencing in our body. It's here that self-awareness is born.

This self-awareness, this complex construction of emotion, moves up to the cerebral cortex, specifically the left insula. Here it collects more information, the logic and memory characteristic of the left hemisphere of the brain, and then travels over to the right insula, where new, deeper layers of emotion come into play. It is here, in the right-hemisphere's insula, that body states (shaking, dry mouth, difficulty breathing) are translated into social emotion (in this case, love at first sight). If you feel happy, chances are you are feeling it in the insula.[16] In bipolar II hypomania, you might feel happy even more intensely.

So there you have it: your brain at work. If you have bipolar II, most of the messages and responses coursing through your brain are dead on—but there is enough neurotransmitter dysfunction to affect the way you think, the way you feel, and the way you remember and perceive situations.

This, in brief, is the physiology of the brain. I hope it has helped you understand the anatomical roots of your bipolar II.

The scientists may say that what makes us who we are all comes down to the way we are wired: the way our neurotransmitters "talk" to each other and the amount of brain chemicals that are released or not released. It is the chemicals talking

• DOES A VIRUS CAUSE BIPOLAR DISORDER?

Whenever we eat an exotic food, somehow it always tastes like chicken. Similarly, whenever we are trying to find the cause of a disease, more than one theory declares it a virus. But in this case, a virus actually could very well be behind bipolar disorder. A neurotrophic virus (one that affects the central nervous system) called Borna disease virus (BVD) has been found to affect animal behavior and may affect humans as well. An article by Robert Kunzig in *Discover* describes how a horse with BVD would stand lethargic, his head down, then he'd suddenly start walking around in circles, smaller and smaller, only to stop abruptly and stand still again; he'd refuse to eat. He would exhibit behavior more and more erratic, banging his head against his stable wall and gnashing his teeth. Unfortunately for horses, a BVD infection usually meant they'd end up dead—from a fractured skull or malnutrition.[17]

Scientists in Germany have determined that BVD is present in humans and that, rather than killing them, it affects the way they think. We very well might be born with this virus clinging to one of our DNA strands; it may lie dormant for years or for a lifetime, but if it is activated, our bodies may not reject it. Instead, the virus may affect the chemicals in our brain, causing certain affective disorders, such as depression—and bipolar disorder.[18]

There hasn't been enough research on the BVD connection, but an antiviral agent commonly prescribed in Europe, amantadinesulfate, has been found to work effectively in humans who have both depression and the BVD virus.[19]

when we are depressed or anxious, when we have trouble sleeping, if we tend to gain weight, if yellow makes us feel sunny, if blue makes us dreamy, if peanuts make us sneeze—it is these chemicals, with their unemotional names that largely govern how and when we experience emotions.

But as real as our physiology is, as truly as it enables us to test and understand emotion, there is another "E word" too: environment. Chemicals don't exist in a vacuum; situations can make a neurotransmitter active, triggering a gene that's been quiet for years or even decades. Nurture, along with your family's genetic structure and history, is the topic of the next chapter in the story of how bipolar II takes hold of us and doesn't let us go.

6

Personality and Family History

> Think of the capacity to learn! The fresh-
> ness, the temperament, the will of a baby a
> few months old!
>
> —MAY SARTON

IT WASN'T AS if my Great Uncle Meyer had any great love for
horses. It was just the opposite. The last time he saw a live horse
was when it held a Russian Cossack on its back, a few months
before he and the rest of his family fled to America and ended
up in Brooklyn.

Meyer had a particularly sunny disposition. To this day, I hear
stories about him, how he had laughed and charmed the crowd,
how he had the biggest heart in all the world and you couldn't
help but love him.

One afternoon, I'm told (I imagine it cold, rainy, and bleak,
with dirty puddles lining the narrow city street), Meyer was
coming home from school when he saw the horse. In those
days, the police did their rounds on horses. When they needed a

break, they'd hitch their horses to a post and stop in at a local eatery.

Normally, Meyer wouldn't see a thing. It would be like noticing the old women who were always sitting on the chairs they brought outside, or like noticing the pigeons that gathered around the Yugoslavian's hot-chestnut cart. But for some reason, maybe because he himself was wet and cold, Meyer noticed this horse. It was shivering, as the drenched saddle dripped water down its haunches. There was blood around its muzzle, as if it had been trying for too long to pull away from its reins. While Meyer watched, the rain falling down his cap and into his eyes as well, the horse lifted its head and shook off the water that had flattened its mane. He heard it utter a small neigh, more of a groan than a horse sound.

That alone might have riveted my Uncle Meyer, but what made him take action were the eyes. One look at those enormous brown eyes, flecked with bloodspots, water dripping down the lids, and he almost stopped breathing. He tentatively put his hand on the slope of its nose. It was soft, like sweaty suede, the nostrils ice cold. Where was the policeman? Meyer looked around and couldn't find anyone.

So what was he to do? Just as he would if he found a stray puppy on the street, Meyer wanted to take the horse home. He unlooped the reins from around the lamppost. He took his coat off and put it over the horse's broad back; it was just big enough to cover the saddle. He took the reins and started to move away. "Giddup," he said, then clicked his tongue. That's how he'd heard it done on the radio. "Giddup." The horse lifted up its head, shook its mane again, and then started to walk with Meyer. He could barely hear its footfalls, the rain was falling so fast.

Despite the cold, Meyer had started to sweat underneath his cap. He took it off and stuffed it into his coat pocket. When he got to his tenement's front door, he pulled it open and, using his outstretched foot, eased the horse into the small foyer. "Come on, just a little bit more." The horse swallowed up the whole space. "Good boy."

The horse snorted and lifted his head, pulling at the reins. Uncle Meyer was almost lifted from the floor. "Whoooaa."

He turned the horse toward the narrow stairway. He could hear Mrs. Stein clanging dishes in her first-floor apartment. He could hear Mr. Olden's phlegmy cough. A single light bulb lit his way up the stairs.

Uncle Meyer stayed to the right of the horse, and slightly in front. He tried to protect it from falling as they slowly climbed the tenement stairs. His family lived on the fifth floor. Each floor had a small landing where Meyer would rest with the horse. He tried to dry its face with the now soaking coat. On the third floor, breathing hard, Uncle Meyer looked right at the horse and told it, "Almost home." The Feinberg kids were shouting at each other in the nearby apartment. The new baby wailed.

As Meyer approached the fifth floor, he could smell the sweet-sour scent of fried onion and chicken fat. His mother was cooking. Good. There would be something for the poor horse.

He opened the door and told the horse to wait, holding up his hand. "Momma," he shouted. "Mom, come here." His mother came out of the kitchen, her face flushed from the heat of the stove, her ankles swollen. She brushed a strand of brown-grey hair from her forehead. "What, my Meyer? What?"

When she saw Meyer standing in the living room, the front door ajar, she almost screamed. "What, are you crazy, my son? Where is your coat? Your shoes, they are filthy. Look at my floor."

Meyer put up his hand. "You don't understand, momma. We have to help."

His mother frowned, the crease between her eyes deepening. As she was about to say something, Meyer flung the door open and there, half in, half out of the apartment, was a horse.

"Eegggghh!" she screamed, startling the horse. It began to twist his head, trying to free itself from the reins. It stomped its feet. It snorted.

"Eegghh!"

The policeman, who'd been outside, following his horse's muddy tracks, heard the scream. He ran up the stairs, his nightstick out, ready to fight. When he saw his horse, he started to snarl. "What's here, what's goin' on, what are you doing with my Daisy?"

The doors to the apartments, up and down the stairs, flew open. People looked up; they pointed; the young Mrs. Melowitz leaned over the upstairs rail so far that she almost fell. The horse continued to stomp its feet. It whinnied.

Eventually the policeman was able to get his Daisy back down the stairs and out of the tenement. He gave Meyer a scolding, but he didn't arrest him. "I just wanted to help him. He looked so cold."

"It's a she. And she's fine."

This is my family's favorite Uncle Meyer story, the big-hearted, nutty guy! But I didn't think Uncle Meyer was crazy. I completely understood why he did what he did. One look at the horse's eyes, and I too would have been hooked. I would have done anything to make it look less sad.

When physicians look for bipolar disorder, they always look at a patient's family history. But maybe they should look at their eyes.

The Roots of Semi-Madness

Maybe it was on the boat coming from Russia, maybe walking to school, weaving in and out of the garbage, maybe it had to do with the day of the horse. Whatever the situation that ignited my family's bipolar genes, I believe Uncle Meyer was where they burst onto our DNA scene, grabbed the brain's gray matter, and held on for dear life.

Family history. It plays a role in cardiovascular disease, in a predilection to cancer, and in the color of your eyes. And it makes sense that if someone in your family had bipolar disorder, you would be more at risk for developing it. One of the reasons your familial background puts you at risk has to do with the likelihood of inheriting genes that can lead to the disorder.

Swimming in the (Gene) Pool

We've all seen strands of DNA, or deoxyribonucleic acid, portrayed in everything from medical labels to sci-fi flicks, those curved "ladders" that we're told we've inherited from our family and that carry the blueprint of who we are. It's a difficult concept to accept: these strands of DNA make us who we are? The pattern in each strand dictates everything from the color of our eyes to our predilection for bipolar II? Yes. And yes. Bascially, DNA is protein in its most infinitesimal form—amino acids. The sequence of these amino acids—only 20 in all!—give our cells instructions on how we are to grow, on how we think and feel, and on the way we look. These same amino acids may have instructions to create cancer cells or chemical imbalances in the brain, but it takes an outside stimulus to "trigger" these instructions and make them real. For example, there may be a history of lung disease in your family, but it wasn't until you lit up that first cigarette that the instructions came alive.

Bipolar II is not simply a "watered down" version of bipolar I. Not only do its symptoms demonstrate the difference between I and II, but research has revealed that different areas of the brain are involved, in different intensities, as well as a different genome, or chromosome structure of your DNA. You are more susceptible to any bipolar disorder if you happen to have inherited chromosome 18q along with those that gave you blue eyes or flat feet.

But here's the most interesting part: Although both bipolar I and bipolar II are characterized by this chromosome 18q, only BP II's 18q version has a high concentration of alleles (a "cluster" of two or more genes occupying the same space on a chromosome) at specific locales, or markers, on its chromosome strip.[1]

Thanks to advances in molecular diagnostic techniques, scientists have been able to delve deeper into our genome structure than ever before. Recently, a gene called DGKH on chromosome 13 has been isolated as a "bipolar disorder gene"; a greater proportion of people with the condition than of their nonbipolar counterparts have this DGKH gene.[2] Not only can scientists now pinpoint mental illness to an infinitesimal strand of DNA, but our cells also create "second messengers," molecules that help regulate cell metabolism from conception. These second messengers are responsible for activating particular genes on our chromosomes' strands. When the second messengers malfunction or do not have the correct "activation factor," the gene in question will not light up. And failure to light up certain genes can lead to psychiatric problems. One of the ways psychotropic drugs work is by causing the right genes to turn on, staving off the possibility of a messenger turning on the wrong one.[3]

More physical proof: people with bipolar I and II have been found to have a different distribution of red blood cell plasma (regardless of whether they are Type A, B, or O) and to have different levels of the neurochemical combination dopamine-hydroxylase in the brain.[4]

The Role of Family History

Family history may dictate everything from your risk of cardio-vascular disease to your propensity to gain weight. Those strands of DNA we inherit from our family make us predisposed to certain diseases and conditions—including bipolar disorder. In fact, according to statistics from the Depression and Bipolar Support Alliance (DBSA):

- Thirty percent of children born to one bipolar parent are at risk of getting the disease themselves.
- If both parents have bipolar disorder, the numbers go up to between 50 and 75 percent.
- Over two-thirds of people with bipolar disorder have at least one close relative suffering from bipolar or from major depression (DM).

However, although family history of, say, heart disease can put you at risk, it is not engraved in stone. If you maintain a healthful lifestyle, heart disease may never show up. Similarly, unrelenting stress may trigger bipolar disorder if there is a family history of the disorder.

When I think of the role of family history, nothing says "bipolar" more clearly than Roberta's dad. He made the word *ostentation* an understatement, insisting on an extremely lavish wedding for his daughter.

Roberta's wedding, thirty years ago, involved 350 guests, 8 bridesmaids in pink voille, and 10 ushers in top hat and tails.

Pink roses and pink candles lined the aisle at every pew; the bride wore a custom-made beaded dress of white lace and carried a giant bouquet of pink roses and pale blue morning glories; even the invitations were personalized and painstakingly hand-printed. The food was impeccable: strawberries in champagne, Chilean sea bass, and a wedding cake with eight tiers. All for twenty-one-year-old Roberta.

This entire wedding extravaganza, at the time worthy of a movie star coupling, might have sounded amazing written up in *People*. But Roberta was from a middle-class family in Illinois, and there was no way her parents could afford it. The wedding put her dad over $20,000 in debt (more than "a lot" thirty years ago), but you'd never know it. His charisma and charm hid his problems—and his possible bipolar disorder. He simply wanted his daughter to be happy.

Meanwhile, in the irony of ironies, Roberta had dreaded her wedding. She told me she hadn't wanted to get married, but "the plans took on a life of their own when my parents got involved." She didn't even love the guy she was marrying; she wanted to be out on her own; she wanted to earn her own money. But here she was walking down the aisle with her dad, watching the groom, in his top hat and tails—and white gloves, for heaven's sake!—at the front of the church getting closer and closer with every step. Her anxiety was so deep that she was numb; "I was simply going through the motions." Three years later, she had divorced. Although no one ever diagnosed Roberta's dad as having bipolar disorder, she herself was diagnosed with bipolar II years later. Did family history play a role? All signs point to yes, although there is no definitive proof.

When I ask my relatives if they recall any signs of bipolar disease in my parents, they say no. Nor do they see it in me. Instead, they see *joie de vivre,* a hard-working success, and, okay, okay, some financial irresponsibility, too. But disease? Never.

Family history often plays a role in disease, which is the reason why health professionals hand you a clipboard at your first visit and ask you to answer several pages of questions about your past and your family's past. But bipolar II can be difficult to identify. In many cases, a person with bipolar II will describe a close relative who was depressed—but may not recall any manic-depressive behavior or anything unusual. And if a relative happened to have frequent bouts of hypomania in which he or she experienced heightened energy, increased functionality, and intense focus, the condition is often nearly impossible to detect. After all, when a person appears happy, sociable, and successful, they certainly don't seem to be mentally ill! By the time the cycle works its way into anxiety, paranoia, and irritability, bipolar II begins to look like depression—and that's what the outside world will see.

The possibility of inheritance playing a role in disease was first put forth by Dr. Emil Kraepelin, who was considered the father of modern psychiatry, in the 1920s. Since then we've accumulated statistics and studies on almost every type of disease or condition humans (and their pets) can have, on mothers and sons, fathers and daughters, you name it. We've had studies about twins who lived together and those who were separated at birth. But the crucial word in all these studies is *may.* My father died of a heart attack at fifty-two, but I'm fifty-nine and still (knock wood) going strong. A friend of mine had no history of breast cancer in her family, yet she was recently diagnosed (thankfully, it was caught in time). *May.* Because whether or not you end up inheriting a disease is not etched in stone. Your fate is not just in your genes, but also in the way you were raised. (And even then, it can be a crap shoot.) The family trees are even more ambiguous when it comes to emotional disorders; chemical imbalance may be in place when you were born or may develop over time.

• SOME BIPOLAR STATISTICS [5]

- Bipolar disorder is the sixth-leading cause of disability throughout the world.
- Approximately 3.4 million children and teens who have been diagnosed with depression really have bipolar disorder.
- Bipolar women are more likely to be misdiagnosed with depression and bipolar men with schizophrenia.
- Three times as many bipolar women than men will experience rapid cycling—quickly swinging from depression to mania, and vice versa.

Nonetheless, *may* is a potent word and shouldn't be ignored. Family history can give us clues to disease—and ultimately, this *may* lead to successful treatment. One of the most famous resources for investigating bipolar disorder and the familial connection are the Amish people in Pennsylvania. Because the Amish have an unchanging centuries-old environment, a small, self-contained population (approximately 12,000), and a closed culture in which people marry and have children at a young age, they are ideal candidates for genetic study. For Dr. Janice Egeland in 1976, they provided a "living laboratory" in which she and her colleagues could research possible signs of inherited bipolar disorder. One of their latest Amish studies shows that 38 percent of children with bipolar parents were at risk of developing the disease, as opposed to only 17 percent of a control group whose members had well parents but one sibling with the disease.[6] Another study found a bipolar link in over 1,000 people in 250 families across the country.[7]

• ANTICIPATION

In this case, it's not defined as "eagerly waiting." The anticipation theory in mental illness states is an environment in which a particular family gene becomes corrupted and more dominant in each succeeding generation.[8] In other words, if your grandfather had a tendency to be overly dramatic, your father's behavior might be not merely dramatic, but occasionally self-destructive. And you might exhibit the symptoms of bipolar II.

The Elusive Butterfly: Temperament and Personality

Watch a group of kids playing soccer. All will know how to lace up their shoes and put on their knee shields. Each one will take his or her place on the field, ready to roll. And each one knows the rules by heart and wants the team to shine. The referee blows his whistle and the game begins.

Now watch these kids—and note their subtle differences. Some of them will be red-faced from screaming, ready to tackle head on. Some will be looking around, checking out an insect or rock near their foot. Still others will be smiling, engaged, enjoying the game.

Yes, a lot of their personality is in the genes they inherited. Yes, a lot of it has to do with the home they grow up in. But there's also something else, something that every baby is born with that is neither nature nor nurture. It's called temperament.

In formal terms, temperament is the way a person acts in a given situation. Drs. Stella Chess and Alexander Thomas[9] took this definition one step further and studied temperament as it pertained to childhood development. They demonstrated that every child develops a specific temperament, recognizable within a few weeks after birth, which has no correlation with environment and psychological development. To the surprise of many therapy patients, mothers, though much maligned in some periods of the history of the study of child development, are not totally responsible for their children's mental disorders.[10] The three major categories that Chess and Thomas constructed from the studies were the Difficult Child, the Easy Child, and the Slow-to-Warm-Up Child. Newer research, however, has revealed a fourth: the Anxious-Sensitive, or Hypersensitive, Temperament, a personality trait more often found in people with bipolar II.[11]

Janice told me about the time she and her husband Roger started couples therapy. They were happy with each other and planned to marry, but both had been in previous marriages and there were some problems. For example, Janice kept talking about her problems at work, how this one had to be talking about her, that one snubbed her. She was hypersensitive to the core, and, as the hypersensitive usually are, hypervigilant as well.

Roger, on the other hand, was prone to depression. Janice's therapist mentioned a couples therapy study that was going on at a local university hospital; the participants got free therapy with the stipulation that their sessions be video-recorded for the researchers. Janice told Roger about the program, and they decided to try it. They couldn't afford couples therapy on their own, and this was a way to ensure they were "right" for each other.

The first few sessions were illuminating. The psychiatrist was a soothing, impartial guide who made the environment safe. Janice was able to articulate her anxiety about getting fired or losing a friend, and Roger was able to discuss the heavy, lethargic symptoms he had when he was depressed. They were making progress.

One evening, Janice got there a few minutes early. She waited in the hall, not wanting to enter the room without Roger. She kept looking at her watch. Five minutes. Ten minutes. The time for the session to start finally came—and went. Janice felt her mouth go dry, her heart pounding. She was terrified. Roger wasn't there! He wasn't coming. He was leaving her, she just knew it. When the doctor came out of the office to see what was keeping them, he found a terrified, frenzied Janice. She didn't calm down until Roger appeared—only five minutes late.

Janice did not react to the situation in a "normal" way. Most people would simply assume that Roger would be there soon enough. Although she'd been unsuccessfully treated for anxiety for several years, three years after this incident Janice was diagnosed with bipolar II. Janice told me that her mother and father always talked about her being hypersensitive and anxious. Her mother would say, "Janice was born that way."

Is bipolar II disorder something you inherit from your family? Is it your temperament, the personality you were born with? Or does it spring from the way your genetic structure was triggered as you lived your life? The answer is most likely that all three play a part—combined with the way your brain is wired. Scientists do not have all the answers yet, but we can at least make an accurate diagnosis today, even though we can't pinpoint the disorder's cause.

In reality, as interesting as exploring the roots of bipolar II can be, it's of less consequence than finding out you have bipolar II—especially after years of misdiagnosis. In the next chapter, I'll be going over some of the tools psychiatrists use to diagnose bipolar II, and I'll share some of the insights of the physicians I interviewed for this book.

7

Diagnosis

We shall find peace. We shall hear the angels,
we shall see the sky sparkling with diamonds.

—ANTON CHEKHOV

THERE'S SOMETHING ABOUT this quote that gets me every time. For me, it's what I yearn for: internal peace. It's the calm that comes from the certainty of knowing, at the core, that no matter what the stress in your life, the pain, or the insecurity, you are standing on solid ground. It might be rocky, but somewhere in your brain, you *know* you are secure; and this certainty is as deeply embedded and automatic as breathing.

But this quote evokes more than the desire for peace. By the time I'm reading "sky sparkling with diamonds," I am also struck with the passion, the bottomless glory, which seems, at least to me, to accurately describe hypomania. It's as if it's saying you can have internal peace—and still remain sparkling, hopeful. It's like a creative visualization I once tried in my quest for calm. Sitting on a chair, your feet firmly on the ground, you are to feel the energy from the earth going up from your feet to the top of your head; you are "grounded." At the same time, energy from above sparkles from the top of your head to the bottom of your feet, into the grounding earth.

In other words: peaceful, calm, sure, *and* energized.

Gracie and the Man Who Got Away

There's an old adage that everything happens for a reason, and that includes relationships. If someone breaks up with you, it might hurt, but everyone around you says, "It's for the best." She wasn't your type. He was a gold digger. She never pulled her weight. And eventually you agree.

That should have been the end of the story for Gracie, but it wasn't. And it seemingly came out of nowhere. Gracie described her family life as loving, warm, "normal." She had a happy childhood. All went swimmingly for her, and she'd taken a designated path: high school, college, and work.

But in her first job out of college, where she was an assistant to an advertising account executive in Chicago, she met Craig. He was a brilliant art director, very confident, and when he turned a certain way, he looked a lot like George Clooney. A flirtation soon became a love affair, and about one year later, Gracie moved in with Craig.

Another year went by that was pure magic for Gracie. Craig's apartment was along the river; when she looked out from his terrace, she could see the sun glimmering on the water; when she looked down, she could see people walking and riding bikes.

As things are wont to do, however, the situation changed: in Gracie's case about a month later. Craig got a job offer in Houston, a position working for one of his clients in-house. It was one of those six-figure salaries you can't say no to. He asked Gracie to go with him. She was delighted, although her joy wasn't entirely undiluted. Craig had never asked her to marry him, and whenever she brought the subject up, he became evasive.

Okay, so he had a commitment problem. Gracie decided to take the plunge anyway. It would be an adventure!

That's when things started unraveling. With no friends and no luck finding a job, Gracie was lonely. She spent her days in their new apartment, which was in an area of Houston called River Oaks, but there wasn't any river like there was in Chicago. Soon, she was too nervous to go out. She started to stay in, looking for telecommuting jobs. Craig started coming home later and later.

It seemed like an eternity, but it had only been two months when Craig moved out. He woke up one morning and told her he was leaving and that was that. Now Gracie had to move. But where? She'd long ago given up her apartment in Chicago. She didn't want to go home, embarrassed, her family ready with their "I told you so's." And she had the added problem of becoming agoraphobic.

Gracie came undone. Not in a full-blown, manic, "I'm going to jump off the terrace" or "I'll book a trip to Lake Como where I can meet the real George Clooney" way, but in a scared, anxious, overwhelmed way.

Quite simply, she refused to leave the apartment. The first time the realtor showed the apartment to a couple, she found Gracie hiding in the closet. The landlord had to call the police. Gracie had to come home, unemployed, unattached, and unable to function.

The first psychiatrist her parents sent her to gave her antidepressants for clinical depression. The meds didn't take. The second one gave her an antipsychotic for what he believed was borderline personality disorder. No dice. In fact, three psychiatrists later, she *still* hadn't been properly diagnosed. As chance would have it, she was at her local Y trying to muster the energy to work out when she heard there was a bipolar support meeting being held there.

Gracie might have called it "those angels from the sparkling sky," but one meeting later, she began to see a professional who made the right diagnosis of bipolar II disorder. Today, she is well into a successful treatment regimen.

Lana and the River Called Denial

If there was anything Lana knew for sure, it was that she *wasn't* crazy. No one in her family was, and she wasn't about to be the first. OK, so she got a little depressed—she blamed it on postpartum blues after her first baby was born. There were times, off and on, when she had trouble getting out of bed. Whenever anyone in her family asked, she had the flu; she hadn't slept well the night before; she was just a little under the weather.

But the depressions started coming sooner and lasting longer. After a week of getting the kids off to school, grocery shopping, running to the drugstore, and traveling 45 minutes to and from his job, her husband had had enough. He was being stretched too thin, and it was affecting his work. He needed his wife back.

Although Lana wouldn't admit it, she was scared, too. She had to drag herself out of bed by noon; it took her two hours to brush her teeth and get dressed; she was consistently late in picking up her kids from after-school soccer; and she was fired from her part-time job at the library for absenteeism.

So Lana made an appointment with her primary care doctor, who assumed she was depressed. After all, she had all the symptoms. And, after two weeks on the antidepressants he prescribed her, she did seem to get better. Lana had more energy and more drive than ever before. She not only took care of the kids, but she took on a full-time job to help with the bills. She was exuberant, whether the activity was making dinner or taking out the garbage; she was more social than ever, seeing friends she hadn't seen in months. When anyone asked, she just said she'd had a long-term flu and was finally feeling better.

But after two weeks something switched. She didn't start buying out Bed & Bath or anything, but she started to get "snappy" with her husband and her children. She yelled a little too often; she told her boss of one and a half weeks that she had a better way of getting a particular task done. Lana stopped taking the antidepressant.

Only five days after going off her meds, she was having trouble getting out of bed. She started to feel depressed—and she had a new feeling: anxiety. What was wrong with her? What was going on? This time her husband didn't have to tell her to go to the doctor; Lana made an appointment for her doctor's first available time. The doctor urged her to go to a psychiatrist or counselor, suggesting that Lana might have a form of bipolar disorder. She gave her referrals and told Lana that these doctors had excellent reputations.

But Lana was still reluctant. No one in her family had ever gone to a therapist. She was terrified—and skeptical. After all, the antidepressant she'd been taking hadn't done a thing except make her irritable and wired.

As of this writing, she had bought five self-help books on bipolar disorder but still hadn't seen a therapist.

Mark and the Day His Luck Changed

By anyone's standards Mark was a successful man. At 56, he was at the pinnacle of his career. He was a senior vice president of a technology firm; he was popular with his employees and loved by his friends; he traveled extensively; he was an avid reader and an excellent golfer.

Mark was charismatic and inspired loyalty in all who knew him. And if he sometimes went on a tirade during a meeting, or if he yelled at a co-worker in an area where everyone heard or complained about his golfing companion's swing, well, that was just part of him. It was shrugged off, ignored, or cushioned by damage-control. The irony was that Mark hadn't a clue that there was anything wrong or inappropriate in the way he acted. He was irritable, quick to anger—just part of what made him a leader.

About a year before he started treatment with a psychiatrist, his firm was bought out by a competitor. Suddenly, the rules changed. The new powers-that-be didn't like Mark's maverick style; they frowned at his idiosyncrasies. It wasn't long into the new regime when Mark got his first warning notice. Soon that warning turned into three and he was close to getting fired.

Mark was puzzled by the criticisms; he didn't understand why management was doing this to him. After all, he had skills and talent that were assets to the company; he should be appreciated and rewarded—not criticized and threatened.

When he yelled at a co-worker by the coffee machine, the new executives looked on in horror. When he interrupted them during a meeting with one of his ideas, they thought him not only rude but too aggressive. When he took a client to a four-star restaurant, they thought him pretentious and overly extravagant.

Mark's predicament drove him into therapy where, even in recounting the stories of the day or the week, he didn't see where perhaps he had done wrong. What was wrong with these people?

In fact, he told his therapist that he was going to write a letter to his new boss expressing his feelings. The therapist heartedly encouraged him not to do it. He said that Mark's new boss would see it as insubordination—and a personal attack.

Mark figured that, yes, his new boss could see it that way, but it would be better to get things out in the open. Mark truly felt like a victim, undervalued and undermined.

Fortunately, after several sessions, the therapist prevailed. Mark didn't send the letter. Although it was still difficult for him to see, he realized that his actions were based on erroneous feelings of entitlement and overconfidence—two characteristics of hypomaniac bipolar II. Rather than writing something he couldn't take back, Mark began working with his therapist on day-to-day strategies he could use to adapt to the new organizational culture.

Subtle and erratic, bipolar II is difficult to diagnose. In most cases, as you well know, it is diagnosed as the disease of last resort, the condition applied when treatment for everything else—from clinical depression to ADHD—is found wanting.

But being proactive about the disorder—gathering information about your symptoms on the web, checking in with your doctor, talking to other people—can help make the correct diagnosis emerge sooner. And more good news: researchers are becoming more and more interested in bipolar II as a legitimate disorder in its own right.

Getting to the Right Diagnosis

If only diagnosing bipolar disorder were as easy as diagnosing, say, a broken leg or high cholesterol. Unfortunately, as with most mood disorders, diagnosis is only as good as the psychiatrist in charge.

For a long time, bipolar II was off the radar screen where only clinical depression and bipolar disorder appeared. Period. But just like diabetes, once a one-word disease, has now long been separated into two distinct forms (juvenile and adult-onset type II), bipolar disease is now seen as a broad-spectrum disorder, with a range of different symptoms and characteristics.[1]

Unfortunately for people who have bipolar II disorder, even with this new "rainbow" of bipolar types, it is frequently misdiagnosed. One study reported that 40 percent of people initially diagnosed with major depression (DM) really had bipolar II; it was correctly diagnosed only when antidepressants had had no effect and after a series of rigorous interviews.[2] The National Institute of Mental Health Clinical Collaborative Depression Study (MHCCDS) followed for 11 years 559 people who had been diagnosed with major depression. The results showed that even after a complete history had been taken and numerous sessions had been conducted before assessment, the diagnosis of major depression was often wrong: 3.9 percent had bipolar I and *8.6 percent* had bipolar II.[3]

This incorrect diagnosis is not necessarily the fault of the practitioner. Most people with bipolar II seek help only when they are depressed—which gives them the appearance of being just that: depressed and nothing more. Further, according to Holly A. Swartz, M.D., a psychiatrist at the University of Pittsburgh's Western Psychiatric Institute and Clinic, many of the bipolar II patients she sees do not remember their hypomanic or manic episodes. "This is not the case for bipolar I patients," she told me in a 2007 interview. "Most people with [bipolar I] are able to recall their manic episodes even when they are in a depressed cycle. . . . The amnesia works both ways. Many of my bipolar II patients also don't remember when they were depressed when in a hypomanic state. They characterize themselves as 'upbeat' people who had an uncharacteristic down time."[4]

Added to this complicated mix is the very definition of hypomania itself. Researchers have been trying to find a common denominator for the condition, a characteristic that is most prominent in people with bipolar II. Some call impulsivity the major trait.[5] Studies are also showing that overactivity may be a core characteristic of bipolar II—with or without any concurrent mood change.[6]

• HIGH ANXIETY

Anxiety may affect at least 65 percent of people with bipolar disorder.[7] Understudied and underdiagnosed, anxiety disorders, either as symptoms of bipolar disorder or co-existing with it (called co-morbidity), have been associated with earlier age of onset of bipolar disorder, less effective treatment when the diagnosis is finally made, more vulnerability to substance abuse, and a poorer quality of life than their correctly diagnosed counterparts. Some of the anxiety disorders have been found to affect anywhere from 3 percent to over 60 percent of people with bipolar II—depending on the research study. These anxiety disorders are

- Panic disorder (10.6–62.5 percent)
- Social anxiety disorder (7.8–47.2 percent)
- Obsessive-compulsive disorder (3.2–35 percent)
- Post-traumatic stress disorder (7–38.8 percent)
- Generalized anxiety disorder (7–32 percent).[8]

Misdiagnosis has yet another insidious effect. Not only can it mean years of unsuccessful treatment, as it did for me and many of the people I've talked to, but *the delay can also render mood stabilizers less effective.*[9]

But all is not lost. More and more literature on bipolar disorder is available in print and on the web, enabling people to be more proactive in seeking help. Physicians are becoming more aware of bipolar disorder, especially bipolar II. And finally, there are now more sophisticated tests to help doctors make a more accurate diagnosis from the get-go.

Testing, Testing

Because bipolar II is usually misdiagnosed for years before it is accurately "discovered," your primary care physician will probably not be the one to pinpoint your disorder. He or she may recommend a psychologist or psychiatrist to help with your depression (as I've mentioned repeatedly, people tend to see a psychologist because of feelings of hopelessness and helplessness, not because they are feeling "high").

Making a diagnosis may not be as dramatic as on prime time's *House,* but there *is* a certain mystery to it. Part science, part interpretation, and part a process of elimination, diagnosing a mood disorder can be a rocky road. In addition to taking a comprehensive family and medical history, your physician is likely to order blood tests to rule out such conditions as hypothyroidism (which can mimic depression) and anemia, as well as any possible substance abuse.

A physician may also use a computerized tomography (CT) scan or magnetic resonance imaging (MRI), two powerful x-ray tools that literally show "slices" of the brain, to see whether your mood swings might be due to a brain tumor or brain injury.

Two other tools, positron-emission tomography (PET) and single photon-emission computed tomography (SPECT), utilize both chemistry and technology; they map the metabolic activity

• BEFORE YOUR FIRST VISIT TO THE DOCTOR

- Make a list of all the medications you are taking, as well as the dosages. *You can simply hand it to him or her; it's also a good way for you to ensure you've written down everything on the form you will be asked to fill out at the office.*
- List all supplements you take, from vitamins and minerals to herbal compounds. *Although these are over-the-counter products, they may cause complications when used with prescribed medication.*
- Spend some time thinking about your family's past. Is there any history of cardiovascular disease? Breast cancer? Any other type of cancer? *Planning ahead will make filling out the forms much faster.*
- Jot down any medicines you take on a fairly regular basis: antacids, aspirin, antihistamines. *These too can cause complications when used with prescribed medications.*
- Call the doctor's office and find out the best time (day of week and time of day) to make your appointment. *This way you will be less likely to spend a lot of time waiting.*
- Call before you go. *Your doctor might be backed up and the waiting room can be full.*

of various chemicals in the brain as it occurs. A "tagged" radioactive chemical is injected into the patient, and as this liquid makes its way through the brain's blood vessels, diagnosticians can see what areas "light up" and which remain "silent." The one drawback? These tests must be given while a person is in the midst of an episode in order for any differences to show up.[10]

Diagnosing bipolar I is easier: mood swings can be so marked that even a layperson may be able to tell if someone has the disorder. Unfortunately, bipolar II can be so subtle that diagnostic tools may not work. It falls to the skill of the psychiatrist to determine whether someone has bipolar II. And, as many of the experts I've interviewed for this book agree, it is often only after treatment regimens for other disorders don't work that a bipolar II diagnosis is made.

Misdiagnosis can even be worse than needlessly suffering for an average of ten years. Studies suggest that many suicides that were believed to have been the tragic result of a major depression actually resulted from untreated bipolar II.[11] And when bipolar II is misdiagnosed as clinical depression, antidepressant treatment can actually *make* a manic or hypomanic episode "kick in." It can push a person into mania.[12]

• WHAT BIPOLAR II *ISN'T*

The following conditions can either mimic bipolar II or exist side-by-side with it.

- Endocrine problems (such as hyperthyroidism)
- Neurological problems (such as brain tumors)
- Autoimmune disorders (such as lupus)
- Other psychiatric mood disorders (such as borderline personality disorder or schizophrenia)
- Chronic and/or clinical depression (the most common misdiagnosis in bipolar)
- Reactions to certain medications
- Attention deficit hyperactivity disorder (ADHD), especially in young children
- Conduct disorder, especially in young children
- Substance abuse
- Anxiety disorders (see "High Anxiety" on page 107)
- Flu-like symptoms
- Migraine headaches

Basically, the best diagnoses are made by those experts who are noted for treating bipolar disorders. They can see past the co-existing anxiety disorders, the depressive state, and the joy that masks the hysteria.

Although there are several diagnosis questionnaires that can accurately determine mood disorders and/or depression, tests for determining the more subtle symptoms of bipolar disorder, including hypomania and bipolar II, are scarce.

In an attempt to prevent bipolar from being misdiagnosed, several of the pioneers in bipolar disorder research devised a tool that could detect subtle hypomania and untreated bipolar disorder. Called the HCL-32 (or hypomania checklist), it was found to distinguish major depression from bipolar disorder in 51–81 percent of the patients first tested. It was also able to differentiate between an "active or elated" hypomanic state and one that was characterized as more "risk-taking and irritable."[13] (See Figure 7-1 for the complete test.)

• FINDING THE RIGHT PSYCHIATRIST OR PSYCHOLOGIST FOR YOU

- It's important that your personalities "click." Your first visit will be one of appraisal—on your part. Do you like the doctor? Do you feel a rapport? In case you don't, make sure you have names of other doctors to call.
- Although diplomas aren't always an indication of a good physician, it's good to know where the doctor went to school and, if you're seeing a psychiatrist, to make sure he or she is board-certified in psychiatry (the official board certification is "Board Certified in Neurology and Psychiatry").
- Don't be afraid to ask questions. How many years experience does she or he have? Does he or she have a sliding scale (if you cannot afford the hourly rates)? Any insurance?
- Decide if you are more comfortable going to someone who is the same sex as you, or if it doesn't matter. That too can be a factor in choosing the right doctor.
- If you suspect you have a mood disorder, make sure the doctor is experienced in that area. And if the person you are interviewing is a psychologist, make sure he or she works with a psychiatrist who can fill prescriptions.

FIGURE 7-1. HCL-32 questionnaire, English version

Personal details: Age ☐☐ years   Centre ☐☐☐

Male ☐ Female ☐   Number ☐☐☐

Energy, activity and mood

At different times in their life everyone experiences changes or swings in energy, activity and mood ("highs and lows" or "ups and downs"). The aim of this questionnaire is to assess the characteristics of the "high" periods.

1. First of all, <u>how are you feeling today compared to your usual state</u>:

(Please mark only ONE of the following)

Much worse than usual	Worse than usual	A little worse than usual	Neither better nor worse than usual	A little better than usual	Better than usual	Much better than usual
☐	☐	☐	☐	☐	☐	☐

2. <u>How are you usually compared to other people?</u>
   Independently of how you feel today, please tell us how you are normally compared to other people by marking which of the following statements describes you best.
   <u>Compared to other people</u> my level of activity, energy and mood . . .

(Please mark only ONE of the following)

. . . is always rather stable and even	. . . is generally higher	. . . is generally lower	. . . repeatedly shows periods of ups and downs
☐	☐	☐	☐

3. Please try to remember <u>a period when you were in a "high" state</u>. How did you feel then? Please answer all these statements independently of your present condition.
   In such state:

	Yes	No
1. I need less sleep	☐	☐
2. I feel more energetic and more active	☐	☐
3. I am more self-confident	☐	☐
4. I enjoy my work more	☐	☐
5. I am more sociable (make more phone calls, go out more)	☐	☐
6. I want to travel and/or do travel more	☐	☐

continues

In such state:

	Yes	No
7. I tend to drive faster or take more risks when driving	☐	☐
8. I spend more money/too much money	☐	☐
9. I take more risks in my daily life (in my work and/or other activities)	☐	☐
10. I am physically more active (sports, etc.)	☐	☐
11. I plan more activities or projects	☐	☐
12. I have more ideas, I am more creative	☐	☐
13. I am less shy or inhibited	☐	☐
14. I wear more colorful and more extravagant clothes/make-up	☐	☐
15. I want to meet or actually do meet more people	☐	☐
16. I am more interested in sex and/or have increased sexual desire	☐	☐
17. I am more flirtatious and/or am more sexually active	☐	☐
18. I talk more	☐	☐
19. I think faster	☐	☐
20. I make more jokes or puns when I am talking	☐	☐
21. I am more easily distracted	☐	☐
22. I engage in lots of new things	☐	☐
23. My thoughts jump from topic to topic	☐	☐
24. I do things more quickly and/or more easily	☐	☐
25. I am more impatient and/or get irritable more easily	☐	☐
26. I can be exhausting or irritating for others	☐	☐
27. I get into more quarrels	☐	☐
28. My mood is higher, more optimistic	☐	☐
29. I drink more coffee	☐	☐
30. I smoke more cigarettes	☐	☐
31. I drink more alcohol	☐	☐
32. I take more drugs (sedatives, anxiolytics, stimulants . . .)	☐	☐

4. Did the questions above, which characterize a "high," describe how you are . . .
   (Please mark only ONE of the following)

. . . sometimes? ☐ → *if you mark this box, please answer all questions 5–9*
. . . most of the time? ☐ → *if you mark this box, please answer only questions 5 and 6*
I never experienced such a "high" ☐ → *if you mark this box, please stop here*

continues

FIGURE 7-1. *continued*

5. Impact of your "highs" on various aspects of your life:

	Positive and negative	Positive	Negative	No impact
Family life	☐	☐	☐	☐
Social life	☐	☐	☐	☐
Work	☐	☐	☐	☐
Leisure	☐	☐	☐	☐

6. Other people's reactions and comments to your "highs."
   How did people close to you react to or comment on your "highs"?
   (Please mark only ONE of the following)

Positively (encouraging and supportive)	Neutral	Negatively (concerned, annoyed, irritated, critical)	Positively and negatively	No reactions
☐	☐	☐	☐	☐

7. Length of your "highs" as a rule (on the average):
   (Please mark only ONE of the following)

   ☐ 1 day   ☐ Longer than 1 week
   ☐ 2–3 days   ☐ Longer than 1 month
   ☐ 4–7 days   ☐ I can't judge/don't know

8. Have you experienced such "highs" in the past twelve months?

   Yes ☐   No ☐

9. If yes, please estimate how many days you spent in "highs" during the last twelve months:

   Taking all together about ☐☐☐ days

Used with permission from the Journal of Affective Disorders, *Volume 88. Jules Angst, Rolf Adolfsson, Franco Benazzi, Alex Gamma, Elie Hantouche, Thomas D. Meyer, Peter Skeppar, Eduard Vieta, and Jan Scott. The HCL-32: Towards a self-assessment tool for hypomanic symptoms in outpatients. Pages 217–233. Copyright © Elsevier 2005.*

FIGURE 7-2. The Bipolar Spectrum Disorder Scale (BSDS)

Read the following paragraph all the way through first, then follow the instructions which appear below it. (The blanks are deliberate.)

Some individuals noticed that their mood and/or energy levels shift drastically from time to time _____. These individuals notice that, at times, they are moody and/or their energy level is very low, and at other times, very high _____. During their "low" phases, these individuals often feel a lack of energy, a need to stay in bed or get extra sleep, and little or no motivation to do things they need to do _____. They often put on weight during these periods _____. During their low phases, these individuals often feel "blue," sad all the time, or depressed _____. Sometimes, during the low phases, they feel helpless or even suicidal _____. Their ability to function at work or socially is impaired _____. Typically, the low phases last for a few weeks, but sometimes they last only a few days _____. Individuals with this type of pattern may experience a period of "normal" mood in between mood swings, during which their mood and energy level feels "right" and their ability to function is not disturbed _____. They may then notice a marked shift or "switch" in the way they feel _____. Their energy increases above what is normal for them, and they often get many things done they would not ordinarily be able to do _____. Sometimes during those "high" periods, these individuals feel as if they have too much energy or feel "hyper" _____. Some individuals, during these high periods, may feel irritable, "on edge," or aggressive _____. Some individuals, during the high periods, take on too many activities at once _____. During the high periods, some individuals may spend money in ways that cause them trouble _____. They may be more talkative, outgoing or sexual during these periods _____. Sometimes, their behavior during the high periods seems strange or annoying to others _____. Sometimes, these individuals get into difficulty with co-workers or police during these high periods _____. Sometimes, they increase their alcohol or nonprescription drug use during the high periods _____.

continues

FIGURE 7-2. *continued*

After you have read this passage, please decide which of the following is most accurate:

- this story fits me very well, or almost perfectly
- this story fits me fairly well
- this story fits me to some degree, but not in most respects
- this story doesn't really describe me at all

Now please go back and put a check after each sentence in the paragraph above that accurately describes *you* (you can print this page, or just keep track of your "checks" on a blank page). When you are done, total the number of check marks.

Add up your total of check marks. To that total, add the number in the parentheses below for the statement you initially selected:

- this story fits me very well, or almost perfectly **(6)**
- this story fits me fairly well **(4)**
- this story fits me to some degree, but not in most respects **(2)**
- this story doesn't really describe me at all **(0)**

The maximum is 19 plus 6: 25 points.

Here's how to interpret your score:

19 or higher = bipolar spectrum disorder highly likely

11–18 = moderate probability of bipolar spectrum disorder

6–10 = low probability of bipolar spectrum disorder

less than 6 = bipolar spectrum disorder very unlikely

However, the HCL-32 is not able to distinguish bipolar I from bipolar II. Another test, the Bipolar Spectrum Disorder Scale (BSDS), was created by Ronald Pies, M.D., a clinical professor of psychiatry at Tufts University, to measure the *intensity* of the bipolar "experience" in order to help determine what version of bipolar a patient may have.[14] (See Figure 7-2 for the Bipolar Spectrum Disorder Scale, or BSDS.)

Although we are moving closer and closer to pinpointing bipolar II, there is still no substitute for a psychiatrist who deals with the disorder on a daily basis. In short, the best diagnostic tool for bipolar II is the experience and talent of the psychiatrist or psychologist you are seeing.

It's one thing to suspect that you have bipolar II—but what if the person you suspect is sick is your child? Read on. . . .

8

Pediatric Bipolar Disorder

Be gentle with the young.
—Juvenal (A.D. 55–127)

Lois was already a mother when she gave birth to Sam. Just like his sister, he gave a whooping cry when he was born. And just like his sister, he slept and ate on a fairly even schedule; he said his first words after five months and he started to walk when he turned one.

All went well for the first few years. Sam was joyous, outgoing. "We called him a shark," she told me. "He was in constant motion, all the time."

As is usually the case with developmental issues, things changed when Sam first went to school. It was there, in a structured environment with his peers, that the analogy of a shark grew thin. The constant movement became a distraction. Sam started to pick on kids; he demanded the best crayons, the best musical instruments. When he wasn't running around, he was staring straight ahead, through the classroom windows at the passing cars, or face down, spellbound by the piece of chalk in his fist. The teachers first said he had Asperger's syndrome, a mild form of autism. Then it was a learning disability (although they didn't yet have the specifics). By the time he was finishing first grade, Sam finally had a diagnosis that seemed right: attention deficit hyperactivity disorder (ADHD). He was given Ritalin, a stimulant that has the opposite affect in children with ADHD, calming them down instead of making them more kinetic. The adults around Sam were more at ease; his high-strung, demanding, and aggressive symptoms had been given a name.

But within a few months of starting the Ritalin regimen, Sam got too thin; he refused to eat and was becoming dangerously malnourished. And his "hyperactivity" began to come back in full force.

Two years later, in third grade, his teachers and school counselors no longer thought he had ADHD. Sam had a new diagnosis: severe depression, combined with severe anxiety. He was put on one antidepressant after another as his parents took him from psychiatrist to psychiatrist.

The family, too, went through a crisis. Sam's sister was embarrassed by him; she ignored him most of the time. She resented that he seemed to get all the attention. His parents' lives began to revolve around his moods.

The nadir of Sam's illness occurred when he started screaming at his mother. During one particular unprovoked fight, he became so agitated that he tried to jump out of a moving car.

Lois's attitude was "I don't care what he has. Let's just get him better." Finally, after reading an article in *Time* magazine[1] about pediatric bipolar disorder and contacting her local chapter of the Child and Adolescent Bipolar Foundation (CABF), a national organization dedicated to helping parents with bipolar children, Lois found a name for Sam's illness: bipolar disorder.

Sam started going to a psychiatrist who specialized in the disease. He was put on a combination of antidepressant and anticonvulsant (recently found to be quite effective in "taking the edge off" manic episodes). Sam had bipolar I.

"It's been a challenge. Sometimes it's hard to say, 'It's not his fault, he's not trying to be willful just to provoke me,'" Lois said. "But I get to leave the house. I can go to work. See my friends. Go to my therapist to blow off steam. Sam can't. He has no escape."

As a child with bipolar disorder, Sam has good days and bad days. Sometimes he only has good hours, but Lois will take what she can get. "Sam's illness has exposed me to so many amazing people, people I'd never have met if it weren't for Sam."

———————

For Jacob, it was grandiosity that did him in. His parents had tried for years to have a child, and when he finally came along, it was, well, a miracle. To them, he was the miracle baby, the miracle toddler, the miracle second grader. When he did a fingerpainting, it was more than swirls of color; it was a foreshadowing of great things to come. When he got an "A" in a math test, they were thinking early admission to MIT.

It was natural for Jacob to think he was this genius as well. How could he not? But other people didn't see him that way. When Jacob walked into class, he'd shout hello to everyone and wave; he was special. He didn't see the looks the other kids gave each other; he didn't notice his teacher's frown. He was Jacob!

But over time, the self-confidence turned into something else. He began to think his classmates were talking about him when he'd hear whispering around him; he began to think that everyone hated him because they were jealous of his talent. He began to get anxious, and he was afraid to go to school. Jacob also became hypervigilant when he was outside his family circle. He had to know what everyone was doing (to make sure he'd be included). Whatever *he* was doing had to be better than perfect (to make him feel safe). And he had to be the most generous, the most humorous, the nicest guy around—anything less and he wouldn't feel loved.

By high school, when he invariably got his first B (it happened to be in chemistry) Jacob spiraled down into a depression. His parents started to get worried; they tried to comfort him, but he pushed them away. He started yelling at them, telling them he wished he'd never been born. He became so sure that everyone hated him that he was afraid to leave the house. All he wanted to do was sleep. He felt better only at night, when he was watching television with his parents. Jacob's parents made an appointment with the school psychologist but canceled when, just like that, Jacob woke up his old "hyper" self. He was wired, unable to slow down; he did his homework as soon as he came home and then stayed up half the night playing video games. But he laughed a lot, he had an appetite, and he seemed happy.

His parents, however, were still concerned. Although he no longer stayed in bed all day, Jacob was irritable and anxious. He had temper tantrums at the drop of a hat. And then, after he'd screamed, say, that he hated chicken and had thrown his plate on the floor, he'd go into his room and cry. Up and down—all in the same day! Jacob wasn't happy. But he didn't fit the model for depression either. His anxiety, his hyperactivity, and his temper tantrums grew worse. Was there a family history of bipolar? Was it congenital, existing before he was even born?

In my case, there were signs, all of which went unnoticed because no one knew much about manic-depression (let alone bipolar II) back then, except that only "crazy" people had it and you took lithium to feel better. When I was in sixth grade, my parents gave me a locket with a tiny full-color picture of the Eiffel Tower in it, which they'd bought on vacation in Paris. I adored this locket, its miniature drawing and the thin 14-carat gold chain I wore around my neck. I'd touch the picture, holding it in a fist whenever I became anxious, whenever the kids at school made fun of me. It became a talisman of sorts.

One morning, I used the hall pass to go to the bathroom. When I went to wash my hands, I noticed the locket was missing. Gone. I started screaming. A teacher down the hall raced in; others followed right behind her, including the principal. In between gulps and sobs, I managed to tell them that I'd lost this special locket, this beautiful present my parents had given me. They tried to calm me down, but it was no use. I was beside myself. I continued to scream. My cries became frantic, and my mother had to come to school to take me home. So desperate was my need to get the locket back that the janitor put a "Do Not Enter" sign on the girls' room and actually pulled apart the radiator, disconnected the pipes under the sink, and even checked the toilets. No one ever did find the locket. The school chalked it up to my being high-strung. Ten years later, they might have called this adverse emotional reaction an episode of ADHD. Fifteen years later, it might be have been thought to reflect depression, separation anxiety, or a learning disorder. Only within the last two years might my behavior have been given its real name: bipolar disorder. But by then I was fifty, and my years of believing a necklace could protect me were long gone. Funny, though, I still remember that locket. I loved it.

Once upon a time, health professionals believed that signs of bipolar disorder did not exist until an individual was around eighteen. We now know that signs of the disease can be seen in children as young as one or two years old. Indeed, pediatric bipolar disorder has become such a hot topic now that it's graced the cover of *Time*[1] and has been featured in many publications. There now are organizations with thousands of members created specifically for the under-thirteen bipolar set and their parents. Because if bipolar disorder can be caught early enough, it may be possible to prevent it from getting worse.

Is Your Child Bipolar?

Statistics show that approximately a million children are suffering from bipolar disorder. One-third of all children diagnosed with ADHD may have a bipolar disorder instead, and according to the American Academy of Child and Adolescent Psychiatry, another one-third of the 3.4 million children diagnosed with depression will eventually be diagnosed as bipolar—and some researchers put that number closer to one-half![2]

If you've been having more and more difficulty with your child over several months, it is possible that he or she has bipolar disorder. But it is equally possible that he or she is suffering from a different mood disorder or is simply acting on the "higher end" of normal. Look over the statements in Figure 8-1 and see how many of them sound like your child (from toddler to puberty). If you find more than twenty to be true, it's possible that your child has early-onset bipolar disorder and you should seek professional advice.

A Profile of the Bipolar Child

Yes, children vary in the same way adults do. One child may be overly bossy and another may still wet his bed; one child may

FIGURE 8-1. Do You Think Your Child May Have Bipolar Disorder?[3]

My child:

1. has a terrible time with separation anxiety
2. explodes into a rage at the slightest provocation (your saying she can't stay up another hour)
3. has mood swings that change several times a day; one minute he's happy, and a half-hour later he's crying
4. is very impulsive
5. is hypersensitive to those around him
6. can't sit still!
7. craves carbohydrates
8. acts very grandiose—she needs center stage at all times
9. is very irritable
10. is easily distracted
11. has low self-esteem
12. has trouble waking up in the morning
13. is anxious in social situations
14. is overly sensitive to his environment
15. wets his bed, although he's over eight years old
16. speaks too rapidly—it's hard to understand what she is saying
17. has a learning disability
18. is very bossy with her friends
19. lies a lot
20. goes on eating binges
21. comes from a family with a history of mood disorders
22. threatens others
23. has night terrors
24. is obsessive and possessive
25. has problems with organization
26. has tantrums that last for hours
27. is too fascinated with sex for his age
28. is too fascinated with violence and gore
29. can't remember things that happened only a day or two ago
30. jumps from one topic to another—her thoughts race
31. sees things that aren't there when manic
32. suffers from a great many aches and pains when depressed

talk too fast and another may have problems organizing her homework. There are, however, four characteristics that nearly all bipolar children share.

Poor Sleep Patterns

Most children with bipolar disorder have trouble waking up in the morning, mainly because they had a hard time going to sleep the night before. They'll shuffle to school, irritated and groggy, but will come to life after 11 A.M. and be fully "charged" by 4 P.M. Children with bipolar disorder tend to be "night owls," and when they don't have to wake up early for school, they often sleep until late afternoon.

And, when these kids do sleep, their rest is often combined with night-terrors, teeth-grinding, sleep-walking, and bed-wetting.[4]

Rapid Cycling

This is where adult and childhood bipolar disorders part ways. The DSM-IV describes a manic or hypomanic state as lasting for at least four days. Yes, that's true for adults, but up to 70 percent of children with bipolar disorder have mood swings—and the accompanying lethargy or energy—several times during the same day.[5]

Executive Dysfunction — From Making Decisions to Paying Attention

When I was in second grade, our teacher made a great fuss about showing us how to write with correct penmanship. She would painstakingly write capital and lower-case letters on a blackboard where three horizontal guidelines had been drawn in advance. Each capital letter extended from the top line to the very bottom line, and each lower-case letter extended from the middle line to the bottom. Hanging letters, such as lower-case "g," had to go just a tiny bit under the third line (an arbitrary issue since it was the teacher who determined whether the tail of the "g" was drawn correctly). The letters had to align exactly with the lines, nothing over and nothing below. I remember trying and trying to get it right (write?) but I couldn't do it. My "C's" and "a's" just didn't cut it. My other classmates would be outside, playing ball and laughing, using their recess as quality time, while I sat at my name-carved desk, pen in hand, trying to write my name.

It doesn't surprise me that one of the common characteristics of children with bipolar is an inability to write legibly. (See Chapter 5 for more information on executive function.) They also have difficulty with other aspects of learning, such as

- Putting numbers or words in sequence
- Short-term memory, forgetting, say, "9 × 2 = 18" in the middle of their "9's" multiplication table
- Creating lists
- Organizing thoughts and activities (which can be especially demoralizing when a child reaches middle school and has to learn how to write an essay)[6]

Attributes Unlike Those of Adults

Children in a manic cycle of bipolar disorder may become a lot more irritable than their adult counterparts. They may also be more likely to suffer psychotic episodes, such as seeing people and things that aren't there or hearing voices or noises that no one else hears. When they are in a depressive state, their symptoms may lean toward aches and pains and feeling sick; they display more physical symptoms than adults.[7]

• WHAT'S THE MATTER WITH KIDS TODAY?

Children and teenagers have special challenges that adults don't. Peer pressure is extremely important to kids; if their friends are drinking or doing drugs, they will be hard pressed to say "no." But what might be so-called recreational to healthier kids is anathema to those with bipolar. Any mood-altering drug will have a tenfold effect on a child with bipolar disorder.

Noncompliance is another big issue with kids. Who wants to take a medication that will make them gain weight? Or make them break out? I wasn't exactly jumping for joy when I saw that the medications that helped calm me packed on the pounds. But as an adult, I was able to make a choice. Kids don't and can't always reflect on the long-term consequences of their decisions. Impulsive and susceptible, they will see only what's in front of them now.

Parents who suspect their child is bipolar should become careful observers, watching and recording his or her moods at particular times of day, his or her sleep patterns, and whether or not he or she lashes out at the word "No" or is very irritable. Parents should make sure they have these written observations to share with a doctor when they seek help. In fact, some parents continue to take notes throughout their child's course of treatment, faxing or e-mailing them to the physician before each visit.

What else can parents do? Read everything they can on bipolar disorder. Join support groups. Be accessible. Inform the school so teachers will know what to expect. And remember that children with bipolar disorder can come off as "adorable" and "charming" during an initial visit with a physican. Make sure to schedule two or three visits in order to get a more accurate diagnosis.

Bipolar Disorder and Its "Partners"

Some physicians and researchers think that pediatric bipolar disorder is merely the latest "disease du jour"; in other words, they believe it is overdiagnosed. Others, such as those referenced in this book, believe it is underdiagnosed. The reason for the confusion? The disorders that look like bipolar but really aren't and the disorders that may exist at the same time as bipolar (a situation called co-morbidity) and need to be treated concurrently. The most common disorders that either mimic or may exist along with pediatric bipolar are

- Attention deficit hyperactivity disorder (ADHD)
- Separation anxiety
- Juvenile diabetes
- Mononucleosis
- Viral pneumonia
- Epilepsy
- Iron-deficiency anemia
- Brain tumors
- Asperger's syndrome
- Lyme disease
- Hyperthyroidism
- Cushing disease
- Clinical depression
- Generalized anxiety disorder
- School phobia
- Conduct disorder
- Juvenile obsessive-compulsive disorder
- Tourette's syndrome
- Substance abuse[8]

The Role of Anxiety in the Bipolar Child

Like two sides of the same coin, anxiety and bipolar disorder are closely linked. In my case, anxiety became my mania. In other cases, anxiety may be present as an impending and unsettling feeling, even as, for example, a bipolar adult spends money he doesn't have or as a bipolar child stomps his feet and screams. Indeed, this underlying anxiety may explain why substance abuse is so high in people with bipolar disease; they'll try anything to feel calm.

Anxiety plays a particularly important role in children because, if diagnosed early enough, a child may have fewer and less intense bipolar symptoms as an adult—or may even recover from the condition completely! In one study, 87 percent of children who'd been diagnosed with bipolar disorder recovered from the disorder within four years, although 64 percent of the children in this group experienced relapses.[9]

Anxiety can also be considered a harbinger of things to come; it can precede full-blown bipolar (I and II) by several years.[10] In one study, 69.2 percent of bipolar adults who were diagnosed before they were thirteen years old also suffered from anxiety; 53.9 percent of bipolar adults who were diagnosed between the ages of thirteen and eighteen had anxiety disorders; and those adults who were diagnosed with bipolar disorder after they turned eighteen had a co-morbid anxiety link of only 38.3 percent.[11]

Here are some statistics on bipolar children who also suffer from anxiety disorders:

- 44 percent also have obsessive-compulsive disorder[12]
- 39.5 percent also have social phobia[13]
- 33 percent also have generalized anxiety disorder (often combined with ADHD) [14]
- 42 percent also have separation anxiety[15]
- 52 percent also suffer from panic attacks[16]
- 31 percent are also agoraphobic[17]
- 18 percent suffered from post-traumatic stress disorder (PTSD)[18]

If your child exhibits high anxiety, watch him or her closely and seek professional help. That separation anxiety or panic attack may, in actuality, be bipolar II.

• ANTIDEPRESSANTS FOR CHILDREN?

In October 2004, the Food and Drug Administration (FDA) issued a warning about administering antidepressants to children and teens; those drugs may increase the risk of suicidal thinking. Discuss the use of antidepressants with your physician before beginning this or any other treatment regimen. And make sure your child is carefully monitored and strictly supervised while taking them.

Getting the Proper Diagnosis for Your Child

Perhaps you suspect that your child's ADHD is more than hyperactivity. Perhaps you believe his depression is erratic; he goes up and down rapidly. Or maybe you think her anxiety is more of a symptom than a diagnosis. Whatever the reason, don't push your fears out of the way. Don't hang them up in your child's closet or keep them in the garage by the skateboard. The sooner your child with bipolar disorder gets treatment, the more effective it will be—and the less likely that bipolar disorder will affect his or her quality of life in the future.

Children with dipolar disorder usually have more rapid cycling. In fact, 70 percent of such children have mood swings that change throughout the day. A new diagnostic test called the KIDDE-SADS is more sensitive to the rapid cycling of children with bipolar disorder.

Yet another scenario: a child with bipolar symptoms may have a deeper neurological or development problem.

What to do? Parents must realize that a diagnosis in children is not etched in stone. Children can change over time; they can have different reactions to medicines as their bodies grow. Pediatric psychiatrists also differ in their diagnoses and treatment courses. As parents, you must trust your instincts; go to the physician you feel can do the most for your child. And above all, be flexible as your child changes and grows.

Treating Early

Children with bipolar II, just like their adult counterparts, benefit from the right medication regimen. But as is also true of adults, some medications can put them in either a manic state or a depression (see Chapter 9). And this is where correct diagnosis is vital.

If a child has been diagnosed, say, with ADHD, his physician would be likely to put him on Ritalin. But if in reality he has bipolar disorder, the Ritalin can make him manic. Antidepressants, too, can jump-start a manic episode. There's been much controversy over giving children antidepressants, especially SSRIs (selective serotonin reuptake inhibitors). (See Chapter 9 for descriptions of these and other medications.) Although some children and teens have become suicidal on SSRIs, the American College of Neuropsychopharmacology (ACNP) concluded, after exhaustive research, that in most cases, suicide or suicidal ideation (thinking about killing yourself) does not occur.[19] Because a child may become hypomanic after being given an antidepressant, physicians usually try a form of talk therapy before heading to medication to treat any underlying anxiety; they also closely monitor the child's treatment. In general, physicians first stabilize a bipolar child's moods and then treat any underlying conditions, especially anxiety.[20]

Another reason to get pediatric bipolar disorder diagnosed and treated early comes down to one of the scariest symptoms of teenagers with bipolar disorder: substance abuse. In fact, the two are so often linked that if someone has bipolar disorder, a physician should look for substance abuse, and vice versa.[21]

Children don't always tolerate medication the way adults do; their metabolisms are different, and their bodies are changing throughout puberty. If you and your physician decide that medication is right for your child, monitor him or her closely. Make sure his or her behavior doesn't change drastically. For example, instead of calming him or her, a mood stabilizer might slow a child down to the point of depression. Any worsening symptoms or aberrant behavior should be immediately reported to your pediatric psychiatrist.

Unfortunately, treating bipolar II in children is not an exact science. We are still learning how pediatric bipolar differs from adult bipolar. There is also controversy surrounding the use of medication in children. The only thing we can do as parents is to get professional help if our children start acting out in very dramatic ways, if their moods switch in a heartbeat, if their schoolwork suffers, and they start hanging out with the wrong kids. We can notify schools and after-school centers about their condition so that teachers and counselors are aware of the situation.

Other than that? Love—consistently. This can be difficult; a bipolar child can provoke even the most patient of parents. Make sure you are taking care of yourself and seeking out professional help for yourself when you need it.

PART THREE

How Is Bipolar II Treated — and
How Can I Live Happily?

9

Getting Help
Medications

The desire to take medicine is perhaps the
greatest feature which distinguished man
from animals.

—Sir William Osler

THE ONE THING that struck me when interviewing people with
bipolar II for this book is how varied our medical prescription
"recipes" are. Some people found Lithium a godsend; other
people, including myself, found it intolerable. Many people
(also including myself) were prescribed anticonvulsants, or antiseizure medication, to help stabilize their moods—but nearly
all of us take a different type. (Just as different designers have
their own style when it comes to making a basic coat, different
brands of anticonvulsants act differently to stabilize mood.)
Many of those I interviewed took antidepressants to help them
in their depressive cycle, but others found that doing so triggered mania and were told to stop. Recently, atypical antipsychotics were added to the mix; these drugs help take the

anxious edge off mania—without the addictive component of antianxiety medications like Valium and Xanax. But just as with anticonvulsants, there are many different brands.

Why one medication over another? Sometimes the side effects of others are intolerable, or other alternatives may be ineffective. The amounts of a particular medication vary as well; dosage depends on an individual's chemistry.

In other words, just as everyone is unique, so too is their medication regimen.

Life in Drugs

It's a fact of life: bipolar disorder cannot be treated by words alone. It is considered an organic disorder, which means it has a chemical base. In the same way that people with hypertension take drugs to lower their high blood pressure, if you have bipolar II you'll need to take medicine, along with making any lifestyle changes that are also advisable.

Another fact: medicines don't usually work the first time out. Unfortunately, most people need to go through two or three different drugs to find the one that is best for them. For one person, it might be lithium. For another, it might be an anticonvulsant. Yet another person might need an antidepressant along with the anticonvulsant—while another might need only the mood stabilizer.

Your psychiatrist should be knowledegable about the different types of bipolar medicine out there, and he or she should be prepared to try different combinations if one doesn't work. And to complicate matters, some people need an antidepressant for their depression and, several months later, need a "trigger" antidepressant to get the original medicine helping again.

Bipolar I and bipolar II can be treated with the same medicines, but in different doses. Obviously, a person with bipolar II will need less strength—although he or she might need a stronger antianxiety medication. Yes, it can be a confusing maze, but with the right physician, you can find your way through.

Once they are diagnosed with bipolar disorder, people usually become medicine-savvy. They can rattle off the meds they are taking with the speed of a teenager's instant messaging. Visit any bipolar blog, and you'll find people discussing what they've taken in the past, what works, what doesn't, even what they recommend. I'm no exception. Over the years, I've been treated with six different antidepressants, five different antianxiety medications, two anticonvulsants, one atypical antipsychotic, and countless vitamins and supplements.

My regimen today? Well, my kitchen counter currently looks like my grandmother's did when she was in her eighties. I take so many different pills that if I get caught up with an article in the morning paper as I automatically reach for each vial, I'll forget what I've taken and what I've missed. It takes a good half hour to count out my pills before I go out of town.

Joan, one of the people I interviewed for this book, took only a small amount of lithium every day. That's it. And she has been doing fine for several years now.

Robert takes an antidepressant, a mood stabilizer, and an antianxiety medication. But I wouldn't change a thing. These are only small inconveniences because *the meds work*. At long last I've found the right combination, at least for now. They are more than worth their weight in counter space.

Obviously, I'm not a physician. I can only tell you what works for me and offer a guide to some of the more commonly prescribed medications used for both bipolar I and bipolar II. (They are usually the same drugs; dosage is the variable.) Which ones will work for you? Only your physician can prescribe medications, so be sure to talk with him or her before trying any medications, including the ones I describe here.

• WHAT YOU SHOULD KNOW BEFORE TAKING MEDICATION

In addition to explaining how each medication works, my psychiatrist also recommends that I research it on the web. He discusses (without any names, of course!) how the medication worked with another of his patients. We go over possible side effects only briefly, so I don't become susceptible to one. (I remember a story about an aunt who read a definition of prostate cancer and was sure she had it.) He recommends that if I feel anything out of the ordinary, I call him immediately.

Your doctor might use a different approach. He might go over side effects in detail—or not at all. Do be prepared for any contingency by bringing a list of questions with you. The ones I worried about the most were

- Will I gain weight with this medication?
- Will my hair get thinner?
- How many pills can I take in a day?
- Will I become addicted?
- Can I drive with the medicine in my system?
- Can I drink alcohol?

Every person is different, so every medical regimen will be different. I remember one excellent therapist's words when I was afraid of getting addicted to my antianxiety medication. She told me to judge which was worse: being nervous and having continual insomnia or being addicted to a pill? The choice was mine. I opted for the pill because the lack of sleep added to my anxiety levels. When things calmed down, I began tapering off.

(See Figure 9-1 for a list of commonly prescribed medicines, including their uses and brand names.)

FIGURE 9-1. Medications Commonly Used to Treat Bipolar Disorder

Caution: This information is for education only and does not take the place of a physician. Please see your doctor before starting any medical regimen, and be sure to tell him or her of any prescription medications, over-the-counter medications, vitamins, supplements, and herbal remedies you are taking, because there are possible contraindications with some drugs.

TYPE	GENERIC	SOME BRAND NAMES®	POSSIBLE SIDE EFFECTS
Mood Stabilizer: Classic	lithium carbonate	Eskalith; Lithobid	hand tremor; dry mouth; altered taste; weight gain; increased thirst; increased frequency of urination; nausea or vomiting; decreased libido; impotence; diarrhea; kidney abnormalities; low blood pressure
Anticonvulsant (Antiseizure)	divalproex sodium, valproic acid; valproate sodium	Depakote; Depakene	*For all:* dizziness; fatigue; drowsiness; nausea; tremor; weight gain; rash; possible liver problems in the long term; risk of birth defects in pregnant women
	carbamazepine	Tegretol	
	lamotrigine	Lamictal	*In rare instances:* toxic epidermal necrolysis
	oxcarbazepine	Trileptal	
Antidepressant SSRIs	paroxetine	Paxil	*For all:* nausea; insomnia; diarrhea; nervousness; agitation; impotence; loss of libido; weight gain or loss; rash; possible liver damage in the long term
	fluoxetine	Prozac	*In rare instances:* worsening depression and/or suicidal thoughts
	fluozamine	Luvox	
	sertraline	Zoloft	

continues

FIGURE 9-1. *continued*

TYPE	GENERIC	SOME BRAND NAMES®	POSSIBLE SIDE EFFECTS
Antidepressant: MAOIs	phenelzine	Nardil	sleep disturbances; sleepiness; dizziness; light-headedness; dry mouth; blurred vision; loss of or increased appetite; high blood pressure; heart arrhythmia; restlessness; muscle twitching; loss of libido; impotence; weight gain
	tranylcypromine	Parnate	
Antidepressant: Tricyclics	amitriptyline	Elavil	dry mouth; urinary problems; blurry vision; constipation; sleepiness; weight gain; headaches; nausea; diarrhea; abdominal pain; impotence; loss of libido; anxiety; agitation; risk of mania or rapid cycling
	desipramine	Norpramin Pertofrane	
	imipramine	Tofranil	
	nortriptyline	Pamelor	
Antidepressant: Other types	bupropion	Wellbutrin	*For all:* nausea; nervousness; agitation; impotence; loss of libido; weight gain or loss; possible liver damage in the long term *Bupropion-specific:* agitation; confusion; anxiety; nervousness
	venlafaxine	Effexor	*Venlafaxine-specific:* constipation; headaches; dry mouth; slight increase in cholesterol; elevated blood pressure
	mirtazapine	Remeron	*Mirtazapine-specific:* drowsiness; increased cholesterol levels; dizziness; dry mouth; constipation

TYPE	GENERIC	SOME BRAND NAMES®	POSSIBLE SIDE EFFECTS
	nefazodone	Serzone	*Nefazodone-specific:* sleepiness; dry mouth; dizziness; constipation; weakness; blurred vision; confusion *In rare instances:* black stool; prolonged erections in men; irregular heart beat; seizures; easy bruising; skin rash
	duloxetine	Cymbalta	*Duloxetine-specific:* Nausea; dry mouth; sleepiness; constipation; loss of appetite; sweating; dizziness when standing *In rare instances:* Liver problems (symptoms include itching, right upper belly pain, dark urine, yellow skin/eyes, or unexplained flu-like symptoms); increased bleeding
Atypical Antipsychotics	aripiprazole	Abilify	high cholesterol levels; increased risk of diabetes; blurred vision; dry mouth; drowsiness; muscle spasms; tremors; involuntary facial tics; weight gain *Abilify-specific:* no weight gain risk
	clozapine	Clorazil	*Clozapine-specific:* risk of rare blood disorder/requires weekly or bi-weekly monitoring
	ziprasidone	Geodon	*Geodon-specific:* no weight gain risk
	risperidone	Risperdal	
	quetiapine	Seroquel	
	olanzapine	Zyprexa	

continues

FIGURE 9-1. *continued*

TYPE	GENERIC	SOME BRAND NAMES®	POSSIBLE SIDE EFFECTS
Benzodiazepines Antianxiety	lorzepam	Ativan	lightheadedness; slurred speech; loss of balance; dizziness; fatigue; blurred vision; memory loss; muscle weakness; risk of addiction
	clonazepam	Klonopin	
	diazepam	Valium	
	alprazolam	Xanax	

Medications Commonly Used to Treat Bipolar II

Lithium

It's not the salt you sprinkle on food, but lithium is a naturally oc-curring salt that can ease mania and stabilize your moods. Although psychiatrist John Cade discovered in 1949 that lithium dramati-cally improved mania, it took twenty years to become an accepted method of treatment in the United States for two main reasons: John Cade, an Australian, was unknown in America, and because lithium is a natural salt, it didn't have much profit potential. One of the pioneers of lithium's use in America, psychiatrist Nathan Kline, dubbed it "the 20-year-old Cinderella of psychopharmacology."[1]

Today, even with our scientific knowledge and inroads into research, we still aren't sure why lithium works. But it somehow acts on the malfunctioning neurotransmitters that are creating manic symptoms and calms a person down.

Lithium takes about two weeks to "kick in," which can be prob-lematic for patients with acute mania. In these cases, it is usually prescribed along with a calming medication. Because lithium can affect kidney function, you need to have frequent blood tests to en-sure that the lithium levels in your bloodstream are safe. Approxi-mately 75 percent of people who take lithium have side effects, albeit temporary, including increased thirst and urination, diarrhea or constipation, vomiting, weight gain, impaired memory, drow-siness, muscle weakness, hair loss, acne, and poor concentration.[2]

Mood-Stabilizing Anticonvulsants

Because of the lag time before lithium typically begins to work, as well as its side effects and its inability to work on everyone, physicians today are prescribing medications other than lithium for mania. These meds are also mood stabilizers, but they weren't produced for the sole purpose of treating manic-depression; rather, they were originally created to help prevent epilepsy and seizures after brain injury. They work quickly to control dramatic mood swings and to prevent them from occurring again. Like lithium, they work on the malfunctioning neurotransmitters that cause manic symptoms. (See Chapter 5 for an explanation of neurotransmitter chemicals and how they affect your brain.)

The first anticonvulsant medication (or antiseizure medication, as this class of drug is also called) to be approved by the Food and Drug Administration (FDA) for use in bipolar disorder was lamotrigine (Lamictal) in 2003. Subsequent research found that lamotrigine worked better in preventing a relapse into depression than in preventing a manic episode.[3] Another study found that although lamotrigine helped people with bipolar I, it had no effect on those with bipolar II.[4]

A side effect of lamotrigine is a rash that may appear five days after beginning treatment, which may lead to a serious and very disconcerting condition called toxic epidermal necrolysis—in which the top layer of skin literally detaches itself from your body.[5] Although rare, it can be life-threatening. Fortunately, there are other, newer anticonvulsants, such as depakene (Depakote), carbamazepine (Tegretol), and oxcarbazepine (Trileptal), that your doctor may try. (I currently take Trileptal.)

In addition to a rash, side effects of anticonvulsants may include dizziness, weight gain, fatigue, nausea, and hand tremors. Note the use here of the word *may*. Not everyone gets these symptoms.

Antidepressants

As sure as winter follows summer, mania swings back to depression. Even if you are being treated for mania with a mood stabilizer, you can still sink down into a depression. In this case, you'll need to add an antidepressant to your "arsenal" to keep you on an even keel.

"Clinicians, particularly during the first contacts with bipolar II patients and when follow-up periods are lacking, may misdiagnose these patients as unipolar depressives," says A. Carlos Altamura, M.D., chair and professor of psychiatry in the Department of Clinical Sciences at the University of Milan.[6] And prescribing antidepressants without any sort of mood stabilizer can flip a person into mania.[7] Researchers believe that many of the people who have committed suicide after beginning a regimen of antidepressants were, in fact, bipolar; the drug lifted their depression enough to give them the ability to carry their suicidal intention out.[8] Offering additional evidence that this may be the case, a 2006 study showed significant risk of antidepressant-induced mania (AIM) in both bipolar I and bipolar II if the medication was not accompanied with a mood stabilizer.[9]

There are four types of antidepressants. (Refer to Figure 9-1 for generic and brand names and side effects.)

- *Selective serotonin reuptake inhibitors (SSRIs)* are effective because the neurochemical serotonin has been found to affect mood: too little of it and you can become depressed. These SSRI antidepressants do what their name says: they prevent serotonin from being as easily reabsorbed into the secreting neuron once it's been "used." Instead, the neurochemical levels get a boost, promoting good feelings. SSRIs have been the antidepressants of choice for people with bipolar II. Sometimes they are used with a different type of antidepressant to help "trigger" more intensity, kind of like the way a good night's sleep gives you more energy the next day. (I take a small dose of fluoxetine, or Prozac, to help jump-start my antidepressant, bupropion (Wellbutrin).

- *Tricyclic antidepressants* are so called because of their molecular structure (three connecting molecules). They are older than SSRIs and are not used as often; they have been associated with AIM and with creating a "mixed" cycle wherein a person is both depressed and manic (read: anxious, irritable, irrational) at the same time.

- *Monamine oxidase inhibitors (MAOIs)* work not only on imbalanced serotonin but on norepinephrine, another chemical in the brain associated with depression. MAOIs, too, are not used often, because you must adhere to a strict diet when taking them: no smoked foods, no soft cheese, no red wine.

- *Atypical antidepressants* are newer. They have a different molecular structure that reduces some of the side effects of the other antidepressants, such as weight gain and loss of sexual drive. (I take the atypical bupropion, or Wellbutrin, on a daily basis to keep depression at bay; the addition of the SSRI called Prozac ensures that the bupropion is working at full capacity.)

How to tell whether a person has bipolar disorder or depression? It can be difficult because hypomania doesn't last. As Dr. Altamura wrote, "Given the short duration of elevated mood symptoms [in bipolar II], these patients frequently do not present enough insight and are not referred to psychiatrists."[10] In other words, it's hard to tell. Andrea Fagiolini, M.D., a psychiatrist in Pittsburgh, Pennsylvania, wrote that the difference can be as subtle as hypomania (the euphoria before mania) and hypermania (the irritability and nervous energy that may come from depression). He believes that people with bipolar II will present the euphoric hypomania, whereas people who are unipolar, or depressed, will be hypermanic.[11] They are wired, restless, and miserable. There's no exuberance or joy—not even for a fleeting few days.

Atypical Antipsychotics

One of the newest medications found to help patients who have bipolar disorders, especially those with bipolar II anxiety, are known as atypical antipsychotics. They have been found to calm a person without affecting cognitive ability, a problem that arises with the antianxiety medications such as Valium and Ativan. They are also nonaddicting, a claim no "tranq" can make.

Unfortunately, the name of this category of drugs can complicate life for patients who take it for bipolar II. About two years ago, my husband and I applied for long-term life insurance. He got a policy with no problem, but my application was rejected. Why? Not because of my bipolar II, which I had thought might be a problem, but because I took quetiapine (Seroquel), an atypical antipsychotic—the drug of choice for, well, psychotics. I am fortunate to have an extremely capable and compassionate psychiatrist, who, at the time, wrote a letter to the insurance company explaining that the dosage I take is miniscule compared to the amount used in serious mental illness. The insurance company reconsidered its decision, a rare occurrence, and I now have the privilege of paying an additional $1,200 in yearly premiums. (I keep my psychiatrist's letter filed away to remind myself I'm not crazy, I'm really not crazy.)

But there's no getting around it. Quetiapine is an antipsychotic medicine, originally used for schizophrenia. Dr. Altamura, a pioneer in quetiapine research, was the first to use it "off-label" for bipolar disorder—which provoked much controversy in the medical and pharmaceutical world. Today, thanks to his work, quetiapine is a typical atypical prescribed for patients with bipolar disorder.[12]

These antipsychotics are usually used in combination with an anticonvulsant for the long term. As many as 90 percent of people with different degrees of bipolar disorder take an anticonvulsant with an atypical antipsychotic.[13] They are particularly effective for bipolar anxiety or co-existing anxiety.[14]

Sounds perfect, yes? Unfortunately, as with all medications, there are side effects, specifically weight gain and a higher rate of diabetes. I know it was very tempting to me to stop taking my medication when I saw the readings on my scale going up . . . and up. But let's just say the benefits—less anxiety without addiction— outweighed the cons. Other people have a real problem with failure to adhere to the drug regimen. Think of it: you're a young adult out in a world where size 0 is the ideal. Knowing that taking a medication that will pack on the pounds is a very real reason why teens—and adults—don't adhere to their regimen. Some of the people I interviewed initially turned to drugs and alcohol instead of meds to ease their symptoms; this self-medication is one of the reasons why substance abuse is so common in bipolar disorder. In fact, studies by Dr. Altamura and others show that drug addiction is a part of the bipolar spectrum.[15]

Antianxiety Drugs (Benzodiazepines)

These drugs literally slow down the brain's activity. They provide an almost instant calmness and can be used to treat anxiety, panic attacks, mania, and insomnia. They are particularly effective in helping regulate sleep patterns in people with bipolar disorder—and sleep is vital to avoid mania. The downside? They are highly habit-forming and addictive and, for this reason, are not usually recommended for more than two weeks' use. If you have taken antianxiety medications for a long time, you'll need to ease yourself off them slowly to avoid withdrawal symptoms.

Success does not live by medication alone. Although drugs are a vital component of bipolar disorder treatment, talk therapy, or counseling, combined with a healthful lifestyle, is also important. Together, these three elements work to make life better, healthier, and more productive for those of us with bipolar II.

• WEIGHTY ISSUES

The stats don't lie. Studies show that 30 percent of Americans with bipolar disorder have developed metabolic syndrome, a condition carrying a major risk of heart disease and encompassing diabetes, obesity, and high cholesterol.[16] They also show that although obesity is a national problem, it is seen even more in people with bipolar disorder.[17] This weight gain occurs because of metabolic reactions in the brain to the atypical antipsychotics—and diets and exercise, although recommended for good health, don't always help.

But science is coming up with more and better medicines for bipolar disorders. An atypical antipsychotic approved by the FDA in 2003 called ziprasidone (Geodon) has been found to reduce the risk of weight gain and diabetes. In fact, many patients have *lost* weight with the drug. "One of my patients on Seroquel had a real weight problem. He also had diabetes," said James Welch, M.D., a psychiatrist with a practice in Ridgewood and Montclair, New Jersey. "I switched him to Geodon and, within a few months, he'd lost the excess weight and his diabetes was controlled."[18]

10

Getting More Help
Therapies

Dispassionate objectivity is itself a passion,
for the real and for the truth.

—ABRAHAM MASLOW

THIS CHAPTER IS the most emotionally difficult for me to write because it involves the help I didn't properly get—for a long time.
Today, I have a great support system around me, including a
therapist I see once a week and a psychiatrist whom I check in
with about every three months to ensure that my medication is
working as it should. But for many years, my coping routines
were more like elaborate "cover-ups": popping a pill to calm my
nerves before going out of the house or pretending I wasn't home
when I couldn't get out of bed. I didn't think about the fact that I
wasn't improving. But the therapists I went to should have.

A Rogues' Gallery

There was the certified social worker who, when I discovered that
my ex-husband had been cheating on me and wanted a divorce,

thrust into my hands a copy of *The Women's Room* (the seventies feminist best seller that forever changed the name of the ladies' rooms in restaurants and hotels) and told me to strike back. When I was too terrified to leave him, she started screaming at me. I saw her at a Macy's in a Jersey mall a few years later; she told *me* I'd hurt *her* terribly.

Then there was the psychologist who told me it was "difficult to have unique parents." My father had died suddenly at a very young age, and my anxiety had increased tenfold with the trauma. When I heard these words, my anxiety only increased; I could never live up to my parents' expectations.

This was also an era, in the late seventies, when people smoked pot as casually as they ordered a drink. Trying to fit in with some colleagues from work, I had gone a step further, taking some "mind-bending" hashish at a party. I ended up with such a bad high (everyone was laughing at me; I was claustrophobic; everyone had either six eyes or two heads) that I remained paranoid long after the drug had left my body and was left with a terrible fear of being poisoned. For about six months I couldn't drink water that didn't come from a bottle. This same therapist, the one who probably had less-than-unique parents, brushed aside my fears. I was just anxious. He gave me a prescription for Valium and called it a day.

The list continues over a thirty-year period: The psychologist who sadly shook her head and said, "Sorry, I can't help you." The clinical psychologist who, in the year in which I experienced tremendous loss (several deaths in my family, including the twins I'd finally conceived after years of infertility treatments), told me I had to leave. The resident and the graduate student who grilled me for three hours at a teaching hospital, checking off my answers on a list. They became angry when I started crying at their unrelenting questions. "This is the price you pay for going to a free clinic," the resident told me as she handed me a box of tissues.

One of the most bizarre experiences I had was with the therapist who insisted I was an alcoholic, despite the fact that I didn't drink more than one or two glasses of wine a week, and who made me, once again, fill out a questionnaire every third week she saw me. I think she was finishing a Ph.D. thesis, but I'll never know for sure. I left after two months.

Introducing the Good Therapists

Yes, the health care professionals I went to back then didn't help me. Part of that was ignorance of the diagnosis and part of it was the misdiagnosing of my condition as anxiety or depression. But today is a brave new world. Finding an appropriate therapist is easier than it once was, especially with the Internet to help you do your research. And fortunately, more and more psychologists and psychiatrists are recognizing bipolar II as a legitimate disorder and are more likely to consider all the possible diagnoses when a patient comes in feeling very depressed.

Talent in a therapist is necessary for proper diagnosis. It's also necessary for successful treatment. Almost every study shows that a better outcome occurs for bipolar II when drug therapy is combined with talk therapy.

I'm not the only one with a "therapist history." Every person I spoke to, right down to the last, jumped from therapist to therapist. The average time it took them to find a therapist who recognized their condition was eight years; some had to wait even longer than my thirty-plus years. And, in most cases, the condition was discovered only after it was clear that nothing else worked, no medication, no talk therapy, no nothing.

Even my dear current therapist, whom I call my Anne Sullivan (after the teacher who brought Helen Keller from the dark to the light), did not recognize my bipolar II for seven years. We worked hard on my anxiety and my depression, but she never connected the dots.

If you think you might be suffering from bipolar II, I urge you to see a professional as soon as possible. Before your first visit, spend a week writing down your mood from day to day. Spend time thinking about your past: Is it possible you have some hypomanic experiences? Were you very, very anxious as a child?

Help is out there—and with bipolar II's newfound recognition, finding an effective therapist is much less of a battle than what I went through.

And then there was Julia. When I interviewed her, she hadn't yet been diagnosed with bipolar II. She'd stumbled across it on the Internet, and the symptoms seemed consistent with what she was experiencing. She'd immediately rushed out and bought several self-help books on bipolar disorder, and she brought them with her when we met.

"Did you ever read this?" she asked me. "Does this sound like me?" The idea of having a bipolar disorder so terrified her that she was afraid to go to a specialist. Her husband and grown children pushed her. Even then, in a room with a well-informed psychologist, she refused to believe it. She didn't want to take any medicines. She was fine; she functioned. Sure, she got depressed. Okay, yes, she stayed in bed for weeks. Yes, yes, yes, she sometimes had so much energy she'd clean her house at one in the morning. She'd drag her kids to the mall and max out her credit cards. In the supermarket, she'd pile her shopping cart with products she'd never use. She was anxious and irritable; she snapped at her family. But, the high, it felt so good! Until, of course, the pendulum swung to the other side. Unfortunately,

Julia refused to believe there was anything emotionally wrong with her—despite the fact that her primary care physician recommended that she see a therapist. Ironically, in Julia's case, it was less about being misdiagnosed and more about complete denial. If she'd gone for help when her symptoms grew worse, she might have been able to spare herself a lot of her anxiety. She could have had a better quality of life right now. Instead, she continues to live in fear, becoming angrier and angrier—and more irritable—with each day.

• A THERAPIST BY ANY OTHER NAME

There are a number of health care professionals who can help you. Choosing which type to consult may be affected more by the provisions of your health insurance policy than by any particular preference of yours. Here's a list of some of the more common types of therapists—and remember, it's not the "type" but the individual's experience and the rapport you share that will make one specialist better than another:

Psychiatrist. This is a medical doctor who has gone to medical school and completed a residency in psychiatry. He or she can prescribe medicines—which is why many people, including myself, have both a therapist and a psychiatrist.

Clinical Psychologist. This health care professional has a Ph.D. in psychology. In the past, most clinical psychologists were Freudian, conjuring up the time-worn image of a patient lying on a couch and talking while the doctor takes notes. Today, clinical psychologists use tools from other therapies to help their patients; they do not administer the same intensive therapy as in Freud's day. Most of them take an eclectic approach, drawing a little bit from this disciple, a little bit from that, in the hope of helping you cope better in the present.

Certified Social Worker (CSW). He or she has a master's degree in psychology. The only difference between a CSW and a clinical psychologist is the number of years of education.

Psychiatric Nurse. This is a registered nurse who can also perform therapy. He or she will also be the point of contact in an insurance company.

Finding a Therapist Who's Right for You

Therapy is based on relationships. You as a patient must feel comfortable with your therapist; you must be able to trust him or her. How do you find that "special someone"? Ask:

- *Friends.* Is there anyone in your circle who has been helped by a particular therapist?
- *Your primary physician.* The advantage here is that the therapist recommended will probably be in the network whose services are covered by your health insurance plan.
- *Your psychiatrist.* Most likely, he or she will give you the names of recommended psychotherapists before you even ask.
- *Members of your support group.* Do you meet with others who have bipolar disorder? Chances are they'll have some names.
- *A local hospital.* A local Bipolar Center would be ideal, but if your community hospital does not have a specific department on bipolar disorder, it will have names of psychotherapists for you to call.
- *Professional organizations.* Is there a particular type of therapy your psychiatrist recommends? Go to its website for a list of therapists who are practicing in your area. If you are simply looking for a therapist who has no affiliation, go to the American Psychological Association website at www.apa.org for a member therapist in your area.

And most important of all: Don't be passive. If you've made an appointment with a therapist whom you don't like or can't relate to, leave. You're allowed to interview therapists; they not only expect it, but they too want to consider whether they can help you.

It's No Longer Just the Couch: Methods of Therapy

Very few people in today's fast-paced world have the luxury of traditional psychoanalysis, where you visit the psychotherapist several times a week and talk in a stream of consciousness about your past, your feelings, your thoughts. In fact, this technique is very rarely used by psychotherapists themselves. Yet, when many of us think of seeing a "shrink," we envision lying on a couch and rambling on about our parents, while the therapist sits near our head scribbling notes.

Today's psychotherapy, or psychosocial management, is a very different animal and there's nary a couch in sight. It focuses mainly on the present and helps change your feelings and attitude with an eclectic blend of techniques. And it can be short-term or long-term, depending on your needs, your financial situation, and the provisions of your health insurance policy.

Does talk therapy really help? In a word, yes. Several studies have shown that when medicine is accompanied by psychosocial therapy, there is

- More time between episodes
- Less need of hospitalization
- Less risk of relapse
- More consistent adherence to a medical regimen[1]

Bipolar disorder makes us more vulnerable to life's vicissitudes; a lack of social support, family denial, life events we all experience— from getting fired to getting married—all create fertile ground for bipolar disorder to grow strong.[2] We might start to drink or do drugs to self-medicate our feelings; or we might stop taking our medications because who cares anyway? We might lash out, creating a more hostile environment that only promotes more decline, and, in a worst-case scenario, giving us an "excuse" to commit suicide. Psychotherapy can help keep us on course.

More proof: In 2007, the *New York Times* reported that, according to a study in *The Archives of General Psychiatry,* psychotherapy for up to nine months is significantly more effective for easing bipolar depression than medicine alone. Indeed, the drugs' success was limited.[3]

Psychosocial management can be much more effective for people with bipolar II than for those with bipolar I. Medication is critical for bipolar I patients; it is the only way they can be regulated. Psychotherapy will help, but the medicine is at the cornerstone. Although you need to take your medications with bipolar II, psychotherapy can go far in regulating your moods and your energy; furthermore, you may be able to "get away with" less medication as your life becomes more manageable.

• HOW MUCH DOES THERAPY COST?

Obviously, cost varies from health insurance company to health insurance company. Usually, a separate division of the company handles coverage for mental health problems. Most plans will pay somewhere between $100 and $125 a session and allow 20 sessions a year. The cost of each session will go toward your medical deductible, so for the majority of those 20 sessions you are not paying full cost.

A new law recently passed by Congress and awaiting presidential approval or veto would give certain types of mental disorders the same physical designations as diabetes and cardiovascular disease. These so-called organic conditions include clinical depression, schizophrenia, mild autism, and bipolar disorder. By being labeled a physical condition, these disorders would not be bound by the mental health restrictions.

Traditionally, the more education a therapist has, the more he or she will charge. Many therapists also use a "sliding scale," with a fee determined by your financial status.

There are three basic types of psychotherapy that are used today to help treat bipolar II. Some therapists use all three modalities in their practice, taking something from "A," and something from "B" and "C." Others are strict adherents to one type alone. Which approach is right? Any of these options. If a therapist helps you feel better, and if you find yourself on an even keel, it doesn't matter whether he or she uses a single treatment modality or draws on all of them like a cafeteria. It's what works that counts. (Please note that the following descriptions are for information only. Only you and your doctor can decide what treatments are right for you.)

• HIGH ENERGY

Researchers led by Athanasios Kokopoulos, M.D., have added energy to the bipolar mix, arguing that bipolar is more a disorder of energy levels than of mood. You can, for example, feel extremely energetic but also depressed. You're wired, unable to focus, talking rapidly. You are far from feeling balanced and may even be hypomanic. But you are still depressed.[4]

Regulate Yourself, or Interpersonal and Social Rhythm Therapy (ISRT)

ISRT is an amalgam of both psychotherapy and behavior therapy. It strives to increase the regularity of your daily routines by utilizing one-on-one, or interpersonal, psychotherapy. Although ISRT has been shown to be effective with bipolar II patients who also take medications,[5] it is only recently that researchers have begun to assess whether this therapy can be used without any pharmacology to help manage bipolar II. Holly A. Swartz, M.D., with the Department of Psychiatry at Western Psychiatric Institute and Clinic, University of Pittsburgh, told me that "Bipolar II itself has different levels of severity." She is currently researching the possibility that people with bipolar II can be treated solely with ISRT and without medication.[6]

The goals of ISRT for bipolar disorder are to help you

- Stabilize your daily routines and sleep-wake cycles
- Identify, track, and ultimately prevent mood swings
- Ease the pain related to a bipolar diagnosis: grief, role reversals, work, and personal limitations
- Educate yourself about the disease

Does ISRT work? Studies show that it is most effective when used as a maintenance treatment; it keeps reoccurrence of episodes at bay.[7] It's also been found to be effective when combined with family therapy[8] and as an adjunct to pharmacotherapy.[9] Dr. Swartz has found it helpful with all of the following types of problems.

Problems related to grandiosity and entitlement. Bipolar II sufferers often feel invincible and entitled. Carl, for example, wrote a review of a concert and spent nine hours mailing it to his friends and colleagues. Jeff, a middle-manager, felt entitled to sit in on meetings with his CEO and was annoyed when his request was rejected.

Problems with regulating mood. People with bipolar II often experience heightened emotion, both positive and negative. These feelings can be so intense that they don't know where to start in "taming" them.

Problems with substance abuse. People with bipolar disorder usually have the disease five years before attempting to self-medicate themselves with alcohol or other substances. ISRT helps diminish the discomfort that causes people to self-medicate.

Problems in recognizing the severity of a hypomanic episode. Samuel felt great—at first. He was productive; his work and his personal life were in a good place. When he got a ticket for speeding, he was astonished: he thought he'd been going maybe 65 mph, when in reality he was going over 100. By examining recent hypomanic episodes and revisiting old ones in the past, patients are able to better recognize that they are hypomanic and ready for a "fall" into depression.

Problems with an inability to remember a hypomanic or depressive episode once it's over. Dr. Swartz has seen many patients who, once out of a depression, call it "uncharacteristic" and maintain that they are usually very upbeat. She's also seen depressed patients who can't imagine ever feeling "happy." ISRT helps people remember that something is different about them, that they do have swinging mood states, and that they must continue to regulate their sleep and their lifestyle in order for history not to repeat itself.[10]

Reality Bite, or Cognitive Behavioral Therapy (CBT)

The basic goal of CBT is to help people with bipolar II use self-monitoring strategies to recognize the relationship among emotions, thoughts, and behaviors—and how each governs the others. Utilizing logic to subdue anxiety or depression, CBT is usually more short-term than other therapies. It is the most studied psychotherapy for bipolar II, and the research has been mostly positive,[11] but CBT has more of an impact if used early in the illness.[12] (Thus it may not be as effective for some of us with bipolar II who have unknowingly spent years with the disease.) CBT is generally not used alone but, rather, to enhance the efficacy of medication.

The best way to describe CBT is using an example: Amy had been flying high; she was getting compliments at work and felt she could do no wrong. But when she was reprimanded by her boss for a minor mistake, the high deflated just as quickly, and noticeably, as a burst balloon. She grew anxious, nervous; she was obsessed with the idea that she was getting fired. She became depressed.

A CBT-trained therapist would help Amy break down her overwhelming feelings into five components:

- *The event.* Amy was criticized by her boss when she'd been "flying high."
- *Thoughts.* This was the beginning of the end; getting fired was next.
- *Emotions.* Amy felt like a failure: "I can't do anything right."
- *Physical feelings.* Amy's stomach hurt; she felt like she was catching the flu.
- *Action:* Go home and obsess about the mistake—creating further mistakes.

It's easy to see how Amy's reactions to the situation were not only unhelpful but self-sabotaging. Her grandiose belief that all was well quickly turned into anxiety, which ultimately turned into depression.

The therapist would help Amy see how she could change these unhelpful reactions to helpful ones:

- *The event.* Amy was criticized by her boss when she'd been "flying high."
- *Thoughts.* Amy had made an obvious mistake, but it was minor.
- *Emotions.* Amy wasn't happy about the mistake, but she wasn't miserable either. It was "no biggie."
- *Physical feelings.* None. Amy felt okay.
- *Action:* Go on with her work and be mindful of that type of error.

The same situation. But Amy *thought* about it differently— which, in turn, affected the way she felt and what she did.

CBT is also used in treating bipolar II to help patients restructure unrealistic beliefs ("I can't lose . . . I'm invulnerable . . . I can take risks because it will always turn out great.") and avoid spinning up into mania.

By keeping a diary and working with your therapist, you can break down potentially vulnerable situations into their parts and avoid spiraling down into a depression—and, at the same time, you can understand that you're mood is moving up the elation ladder a little too fast.

• STEP-BY-STEP

The Systematic Treatment Enhancement Program for Bipolar Disorder (STEP-BD) was created by Gary Sachs, M.D., and his team at the Massachusetts General Hospital Bipolar and Research Program in an effort to determine how effective the different treatments for bipolar disorder were and to help develop a standard that could be used by health care professionals. An on-going program, STEP-BD began with 223 clinicians who participated in the same training. The early results overwhelmingly showed (62.7 percent) that diagnostic assessment was the number-one obstacle to successful treatment.[13] STEP-BD is hoping to change that with a common disease management program that involves establishing a patient's clinical status at each visit; choosing from a menu of treatment options on the basis of medical history, current presentation, and research evidence made accessible to all health care professionals; and negotiating a plan that both clinician and patient are willing to try.

Full Circle: Family-Focused Therapy (FFT)

Bipolar II doesn't take place in a vacuum; it involves not only you but also those around you—your family, your spouse, your significant other, your friends. Family-focused therapy brings them all together to improve the communication, support, and understanding that someone with bipolar II needs in order to keep episodes at bay. FFT usually consists of 21 one-hour sessions, including

Psychoeducation. Improvement begins with education. Your family has to understand what you are going through in order to offer support and understanding. Psychoeducation usually includes a "relapse drill" so that family members can recognize the early signs of either mania or depression and get help sooner, rather than later.

Communication enhancement. A mental disorder does not make for a calm household. Chances are that there are irritability, anger, denial—in other words, dysfunction. This aspect of FFT helps your family members see where they are having a negative effect, as well as encouraging them to recognize and express their emotions about your disease. Here, both you and your family learn how to actively listen, give positive feedback, make positive requests to change behavior (screaming doesn't usually work), and offer constructive, calm criticism.

Problem solving. This area gets down to the specifics, the problems you and your family face because of your bipolar II. Such problems can include financial difficulties, because, for example, you aren't able to hold on to a job. Or they may be social, because recognizing emotional cues is difficult for someone with bipolar disorder, and boundaries may be inadvertently crossed. Or they may be professional, because you need to find another way to earn a living.[14]

The ultimate goal of FFT is to teach effective problem-solving skills to restore harmony in your family, to help you adhere to your medication regimen, and to avoid relapses as much as possible. Studies show that it is a viable form of therapy when combined with medicine and individual therapy.

What about Alternative Medicine?

There are some supplements that show promise in treating bipolar disorder—and others that don't. Here's the lowdown on some of the more popular alternatives out there. Please note that supplements should never be taken in the place of traditional medications, but only as a *complement* to them. Let your doctor know if you are taking any alternative medicines along with what's been prescribed. And *always* check first to ensure that you aren't putting yourself at health risk.[15]

Supplements and Medications

Omega-3 fatty acids play an important role in keeping nerve cells healthy. There is no definitive research showing that this essential acid will help keep your bipolar disorder in remission longer, but a preliminary study at Brigham and Women's Hospital in Boston suggested just that.[16] Stay tuned.

EMPowerplus is a nutrient cocktail of vitamins, minerals, amino acids, and herbs. It's got the bipolar community buzzing, but there are no studies to confirm that it helps treat bipolar disorder. Moreover, there is evidence that it can be harmful. A warning about the drug was released in Canada because it caused psychosis, anxiety, fear, delusion, and even malignant lymphoma; the victims were all taking standard medications along with the EMPowerplus.[17]

St. John's Wort is an herb that has shown promise as a natural way to treat mild depression. But bipolar? Not likely. It's been found to create mania in people with bipolar disorder.

B complex. Studies have found that deficiencies in vitamin B12, or folic acid, may trigger depression; some studies also show that large doses of folic acid may help lithium do its job. If you're going to go the "B" route, it's best to take a B complex because (1) synergy makes the combination more potent and (2) taking too much folic acid, for example, can lead to nerve damage.

L-tryptophan converts to serotonin, the chemical responsible for so many of our moods. And some studies have shown that it can help lithium do its job, as well as treat mania. In 1990 there was a nationwide recall of the supplement because it may have caused, in 1,500 people, a rare disease called eosinophilia-myalgia syndrome (EMS) that could lead to death. It isn't clear whether the manufacturer or the supplement itself was responsible. Better to get yours naturally, in your Thanksgiving turkey.

Serenity is the brand name of a nonprescription lithium. Does it work? According to a study done over 33 years ago, yes. But because lithium is a naturally created substance to begin with, why take something that may not work when the "real deal" does? [18]

Therapies

Magnetic field therapy evolved from the belief that psychological disorders are caused by electromagnetic imbalances; in diseases of the emotions, there's a rise in electrical activity in the central nervous system. By applying strategically placed negative magnets to counteract the positive charge in your body, this procedure is supposed to alleviate the mental conditions. There have not been any studies to investigate whether this therapy works.

Ayurvedic medicine's rauwolfia serpentina is an herb used in India and abroad to treat mental illness, but it may cause your depression to get worse.

Craniosacral therapy is based on the belief that, in addition to the rhythm of your breath and heart beat, there is a rhythm to the cerebrospinal fluid that flows through your spinal cord and brain. When pressure builds up, imbalances in the brain may occur; a craniosacral therapist relieves this pressure via touch. No studies support this therapy at this time.

Acupuncture is becoming more and more mainstream as an effective tool in fighting everything from weight gain and acne to substance abuse—and mental disorder. The technique works by strategically placing needles in your body along its meridian (read: energy) paths to balance your endocrine system. This, in turn, relieves stress, induces calm, and reduces depression. Clinical trials are currently being conducted to determine its effectiveness with bipolar disorder.[19]

Biofeedback measures your autonomic body functions, such as blood pressure, heart rate, and muscle tension, and sends the information back to you. Given this insight into these unconscious mechanisms, you can gain control of them, easing your anxiety or depression.

Hypnosis. Once the centerpiece of a magician's act, hypnosis today is considered a viable therapy for quitting smoking, losing weight, and restoring calm. Does it help bipolar disorder? Because its inherent relaxation alleviates stress, your body chemistry will change and you may become less anxious.

The Feldenkrais Method revolves around a person's self-image; our movements are supposedly based on the way we view ourselves. Poor self-image translates into poor movement, including breathing in and out—which then adversely affects the body and its functions. Utilizing touch at specific points on the body is supposed to improve your movement and, in turn, your body's function. This approach is generally used as a way to alleviate stress.

Some of the people I spoke to were not in psychotherapy; they had either recently quit psychotherapy or depended solely on their psychiatrists and medications. Others participated in group therapy and support groups. Still others continue to see a therapist one-on-one once a week, or once every other week, and also see a psychiatrist. The pattern chosen reflects expense, insurance policy provisions, and time available. Psychotherapy takes commitment, but so does medicine. Taken together, they can help you beat the odds of relapse. I know that first-hand.

11

Living Well with Bipolar II
Making Healthy Choices

To sit in the shade on a fine day, and look upon
verdure is the most perfect refreshment.

—Jane Austen

Kathy had been the kind of person who started planning for the
Christmas holidays early. She wanted to buy gifts for everyone
she knew, not just her family and close friends, but her dentist
and her doctor, her friends' mothers and fathers, the pharmacist
at her drugstore, and the man who pumped her gas. One season, she spent close to $1,000, but she'd charged it all. She was
sure she'd have the money, no problem, when it was due: she'd
get a check in the mail or she'd win the lottery. She also believed
that all her friends were planning a party for her, just because
she was so wonderful—but it was a Big Secret.

Kathy was diagnosed with bipolar disorder after she'd at-
tended a life-coaching seminar that encouraged high energy. As
the two-day event came to an end, she found herself feeling
more "hyper" than usual. She didn't sleep for the next three days;

she had a sense of euphoria because everyone loved her and she loved them all. "I felt like the world was a beautiful wonderland. Buildings and restaurants I'd visited before seemed magical and mystical, like I'd either gone back in time or I was in heaven. I felt invincible and powerful and safe." And then it all changed; Kathy didn't want to leave her bed.

Today, Kathy's bipolar II is correctly diagnosed and under control. However, she'd often find herself afraid of losing that control. That's why she was afraid of taking yoga at first; she thought it would make her feel "too free." She'd been a working actress before her diagnosis, working on roles that were very dramatic, women in turmoil and distress. She decided to change gears, fearing that the acting or the long nights of rehearsal would set her off. Instead she's currently in graduate school with a 4.0 GPA—something she'd wanted to do years ago but never did.

What does Kathy do today to ensure she's on an even keel? She's gone back to yoga but takes it easy, with the right amounts of "challenge and relaxation." She regularly goes to a dermatologist and works out with a personal trainer to help stave off the side effects of weight gain and acne brought on by her bipolar medicine.

"I've also had to let go of certain people in my life," she wrote me. "I was seeing a nutritionist for years, but she kept telling me to get off the meds, and I know that this was not an option. It was hard enough to convince myself to stay on them in the beginning, and having someone else discourage me from sticking with them was not helping."

To help her understand her illness, Kathy also reads books about bipolar disorder, including Kay Redfield Jamison's classic *An Unquiet Mind* and Jane Pauley's *Skywriting*.

———

Jonah's bipolar disorder impacted his work life: "I am self-employed. I have to be," he said. "I can't imagine being able to meet all the requirements a traditional employer demands." Before he was diagnosed ten years after his symptoms first started, Jonah would become obsessive, e-mailing his friends and colleagues all through the night. "I didn't eat; I barely went to the bathroom; I didn't leave my computer for nine hours." He also became hypersexual; he wanted to have sex all the time. He even frequented prostitutes, anything, as long as he could have sex.

But still Jonah didn't seek help. It wasn't until his anger almost got the best of him at work that he realized he had a problem. When he heard the diagnosis, he was relieved. "At last there was a reason I'd been so erratic and irresponsible my whole adult life!" Jonah knows that his medications keep him stable—and so do his lifestyle choices: no excessive sugar, no chocolate, no caffeine—not even decaf coffee because it has small amounts of caffeine in it. He doesn't drink, smoke, or do drugs. He exercises as regularly as possible, although it's sometimes difficult to push himself to go to the gym. But dietary restrictions combined with physical activity have kept bipolar episodes away.

He often opts out of social events with his friends because he feels incapable of being social on that particular night. "Most recently, I had a $70 theater ticket and was ready to go with my friends, but then I faked being sick. I didn't think I could handle my friends, the crowd, just the act of going out." Just saying no is also a part of a healthy lifestyle for those of us who have bipolar disorder.

Does he resent the restrictions on his life? "Sure, I'd rather be able to do anything I want—but the price I'd pay is too high. Being steady and calm is better than a Starbucks latte any day."

If you had to think of an adjective to describe Rochelle, it would be *spunky;* that's the way she describes herself. She was lively and happy and had a wonderful childhood. Her parents loved each other; she and her brother had a strong bond. She lived on a tree-laden suburban street and often played in the middle of the road with her friends. She even liked school and got good grades. So it was more of a shock than anything else to learn she had bipolar II. Yes, she'd always been hypersensitive, feeling things a lot more intensely than anyone in her family. But they'd just say she was being dramatic, nothing more.

Things changed after she graduated from college. She'd gotten an entry-level job at a publishing house in Manhattan and it started out great; she was learning the book business hands-on. But then she met Sammy and was, as she put it, "swept off her feet." He got a job as a professor at a Vermont college and asked her to come with him. Without any hesitation, she quit her job, said goodbye to her friends and family, and moved to New England to be with her boyfriend—who subsequently dumped her.

The pain of the breakup filtered into other aspects of her life. She stopped going to work at her new job at a New England newspaper; she stopped going out to do errands or to meet some potential friends. She stopped going out . . . period. To all, it looked like depression, pure and simple. She didn't get out of bed; she didn't shower; she stuffed herself with Twinkies and potato chips. But she had a reason. Her boyfriend left her!

When Rochelle first went for help, the therapist gave her an antidepressant. But that did more than lift her spirits—it made them get up and dance. She'd didn't need her boyfriend. She didn't need the job. She'd get another one. She'd be a writer; she'd always wanted to write.

When she got an eviction notice, she was shocked. Then she realized she hadn't been paying any of her bills. She also began having a series of one-night stands, something she'd never done in Manhattan.

Rochelle knew she was in trouble and called her family. She stopped taking the antidepressants, but that left her feeling very shaky, vulnerable, and anxious. Fortunately, she was able to come home, where, finally, she was diagnosed with bipolar II.

Today, Rochelle is back on her own again and doing fine. She religiously takes her meds even though they've made her put on weight. "I'm starting to lose it again," she told me. "I'm watching what I eat." The most important lifestyle change for Rochelle involved her sleep. She goes to bed at the same time every night, 10 P.M., and wakes up at 8 A.M. whether or not she has work. "I've missed some parties, but my friends understand. They support me. They know that I need to get my sleep to be healthy."

These three people have different stories, but their lifestyle choices are variants on the same theme: eat healthy, exercise, and get your sleep.

Medication and psychotherapy go far in preventing relapses and keeping you on an even keel. But if you don't change your lifestyle, they will be less effective. Too little sleep, and mania can kick in. Too tight a deadline at work, and you'll be stressed out—leading to mania. Eat junk food, and you'll either spiral into a depression or get a sugar-induced mania.

It doesn't take an advanced degree to know how to live healthy. We all know that sleep, exercise, and healthy eating contribute to a better and longer life. But for those of us with bipolar II, there's another element: stability.

In order to keep your moods in balance, to feel stable and strong, medicine and therapy aren't quite enough. Your lifestyle is just as important a component as taking those pills every day.

Perchance to Sleep

A good night's sleep not only makes you feel refreshed, energized, and glowing, but, internally, sleep restores the chemicals in the brain, such as serotonin and norepinephrine, and rests your body before the next day's onslaught. Researchers have also found that sleep gives the brain an opportunity to organize and store the stimuli it has registered during the day; thus it helps create memory.[1]

If you want to treat your bipolar disorder, you'll need to treat your sleep: not too little and not too much. Circadian rhythms, the internal biological clock that regulates when we feel sleepy or alert throughout the day, and the genes that make up their structure have long been associated with bipolar disorder. When researchers investigated the effect of this "clock" gene in mice, the mice became manic: hyperactive, with less ability or need to sleep, and hypersensitive to stimuli. When these same mice were given lithium, they became calm and returned to their usual scurrying, munching, mice-y routines.[2] Further studies illuminated the findings that lithium altered circadian rhythm, inhibiting those genes that were affecting regulation.[3]

The amount of sleep you get is a good indicator of your moods. If you can't sleep, or if you sleep too little, you may be spinning into mania; if you sleep too much, you may be getting depressed. Regulating your sleep, getting seven or eight hours every night, is one of the best ways to keep symptoms away. You might not turn into a pumpkin, but not getting into bed by midnight may trigger mania. (If you're a night owl, that's fine, too. Just adjust your schedule so you go to sleep at 2 A.M. and don't wake up until 9 A.M.)

• GETTING YOUR ZZZZ'S

Here are ten tips, adapted from the National Sleep Foundation, to help you get a good night's sleep.[4]

1. Maintain a sleeping schedule throughout the week, including Saturday and Sunday.
2. Establish a relaxing activity right before bedtime, such as soaking in a hot tub (adding lavender essential oil will help you further relax) or listening to calming music.
3. Make your sleep environment calming: dark, cool, quiet, comfortable, and clean.
4. Ensure that your mattress, sheets, and pillows are both comfortable and supportive.
5. Keep your bedroom off limits except for sleep and sex.
6. Don't eat anything two or three hours before you go to sleep.
7. Exercise regularly—but not right before you go to sleep.
8. Avoid caffeine, and that includes coffee, tea, soft drinks, and even chocolate.
9. Don't smoke: in addition to the health risk it poses, nicotine acts as a stimulus.
10. Don't drink alcohol before going to sleep. Nightcaps can lead to unsettled sleep.

Build a Routine into Your Schedule

"Routine is anything but boring for me. When my schedule gets off, I start to have problems."

"By keeping regular hours, when I sleep, when I eat, when I come home, when I exercise, I know what to expect. My anxiety levels go way down."

"If there's a special event, like a wedding or a party, I'll plan for it by writing it down in my schedule. Even though it alters my routine, I'll know what to expect."

"Sometimes my friends try to coax me to 'live a little.' But then I remember that without my routine, I lived too much, and it's just not worth it."

These words are from people with bipolar II who have lived with the diagnosis long enough to know that they need a life that's scheduled as much as possible. Routine is the single most effective self-care prophylactic you can give yourself. Scheduling regular hours for sleeping, eating, working, exercising, and, yes, even for relaxing and having fun, helps ease anxiety. It makes you feel stronger, calmer. With bipolar, the unexpected is not always a surprise party: it's a risk that can make you nervous, anxious, and manic.

To get you into a realistic routine, spend a week doing what you normally do, but jot down the times and the activities in a notepad. When the week is over, you'll easily see, "Oh, I go to sleep at 1 A.M."; "I like to eat dinner at 8 P.M."; "I'm ready to leave the house in the morning at 9 A.M."; or "I like to watch TV from 8 P.M. to 11 P.M."

Armed with the facts of your particular time set, create a weekly schedule and try to stick with it as best you can. If you're having trouble doing more than one or two activities at the designated time, revise the schedule until it's exactly right for you.

Staples and other stationery stores all sell appointment calendars. Or, if you'd prefer, simply copy the blank schedule in Appendix A that I created for myself. I've found it difficult to find schedules that don't have a designated year, so I made my own. You can also find blank schedules online or in your Excel program, which will enable you to download a blank schedule to your PDA or BlackBerry.

Diet and Exercise:
They're More Important Than You Think

Yes, we've all heard it a thousand times before: eat a diet rich in fruits and vegetables; eat whole grains instead of white flour; stay away from red meat and saturated fats; and while you're at it, exercise for thirty minutes at least five times a week. Making these lifestyle changes can help reduce the stress levels associated with bipolar II anxiety; they help keep you on an even keel.

I know I've heard this mantra so often that the words have lost meaning. This knowledge alone didn't motivate me to stay on a healthy diet and fitness program.

But here are some additional facts that *did* get me on the "straight and slimmer":

- Lithium packs on the pounds more than other mood stabilizers. In research done on medication used for maintenance over an eighteen-month period, people who took lithium gained significantly more weight than people who were taking the anticonvulsant lamotrigine, with the most dramatic weight increases occurring in those who were already obese (with a body mass index, or BMI, higher than 30).[5]
- Almost every medication for bipolar disorder is associated with weight gain and, in most cases, this weight gain is occurring in adults who are already overweight. Research shows that with every increase in BMI, the risk goes up for obesity-related diseases, including arthritis, cardiovascular disease, stroke, and diabetes. But hear this: *a study maintained over a thirty-year period*

found that the benefits of medications for bipolar patients clearly justified the risks.[6]

- Studies show that when people with mental disorders participate in aerobic activity, they are less likely to become depressed, now and in the future.[7]

The evidence is clear: when you take medications for bipolar disorder, you are very likely to gain weight. Researchers don't yet understand why, but balancing the chemicals in the brain seems to change our metabolism, causing weight gain. But the amount you gain is more in your control than you might think. You might not be able to lose ten pounds before that wedding in five weeks, but you can avoid *gaining* ten pounds if you adhere to a diet and exercise regimen. Studies also show that after several months, the weight gain tapers off; you won't be able to lose weight easily, but you won't be gaining either.

Healthy Eating for a Healthy Life

Eating healthy doesn't mean eating as much healthful foods as you want. Even those Whole Foods all-organic, preservative-free entrées can get you fat if you eat enough of them. But meager portions will make you hungry—and irritable; crash diets disrupt your routine and create havoc with your moods. What works for me is a modified Weight Watchers diet, between 1,200 and 1,600 calories daily, that is rich in

Whole grains, such as bran cereal and whole wheat pasta
Fruits and vegetables—choose what's in season
Healthful sources of protein, such as chicken, fish, and eggs
Low- or no-fat dairy products, such as yogurt, cottage cheese, and milk

Healthful fats, such as olive oil, which increases HDL cholesterol (the good one that vacuums up any LDL, or bad, cholesterol that's been hanging around on your artery walls)

To help keep you motivated, try these tips. They worked for me and for many of the people I interviewed. They might work for you as well.

- An "indulgence allowance" once or twice a week to keep deprivation at bay; sometimes it's a fattening dessert, sometimes it's as simple as a bagel.
- *Keep your sugar off the table.* Although there's no direct causal link between sugar and diabetes, refined sugar will mess up your blood sugar levels—which means your moods can rise and fall precipitously. Sugar can lead to weight gain . . . which can lead to diabetes.
- *Avoid caffeine, alcohol, and drugs.* Caffeine-laced drinks may keep you up at night. Alcohol and drugs can interfere with the medications you are taking; they can make them less effective or downright dangerous.

Exercise Your Bikes (or Any Other Physical Activity)

Aerobic exercise, the kind that gets your heart pumping, accelerates your metabolism; you'll be burning calories instead of eating them. Because many medications for bipolar disorder slow your metabolism (thus keeping hypomanic anxiety at bay), exercise will at least help prevent that slow metabolism from getting sluggish—and help keep your weight gain under control.

The hardest part of exercising is putting on your sneakers. Once you're out the door, the rest gets easy. Although we know how good exercise is for our bodies and our minds, we always seem to resist it: "I'm too tired." "My favorite TV show is on." "I have too much to do." "I have to feed the cat."

But if you *schedule in* your exercise, it'll be there in black and white, staring you in the face, your excuses gone by the wayside. Here are some tips for bringing physical activity—and a better mood, a leaner body, and a healthier heart—back into *your* life.

Find something you like. This sounds easier than it really is. A lot of people think they have to spend thirty minutes on the treadmill or in a step class because, well, that's exercise. Wrong. Anything that gets your heart pumping is considered aerobic exercise and if it's something you enjoy, you'll actually do it!

I'm partial to dance classes, such as NIA, West African, and cardio jazz. Spinning classes are also terrific; you become one with the music. And don't think you have to be Lance Armstrong. People have this idea that spinning is only for advanced exercisers. Not true. You go at your pace, at your level of resistance, the whole time. Nobody's watching.

(If, like Kathy in the beginning of this chapter, you feel that some exercise may make you feel too free, and that scares you, there are structured alternatives that also work: jazzercise gives you dance, but with very structured movements; cardio kickboxing is all about routine and releasing tension; walking outside puts you in control because you decide where to go and for how long.)

Start small. Agreed: you're not going to run a marathon your first time out. But studies show that just ten minutes a day can improve your cardiovascular health.[8] Schedule in ten minutes, say, before dinner or when you first wake up. Get used to that, and you'll find yourself increasing the time—willingly.

Have your gear accessible. Don't make it even harder to get out the door. Make sure your sneakers and exercise gear are packed in a gym bag or laid out on the chair (not the treadmill). You won't even have time to think you don't want to do it.

Add some strength training. These nonaerobic (anaerobic) exercises might not help your mood as much as the exercise that gets your heart pumping, but they can help you maintain strong bones and tone your body (a toned body looks thinner). There are many classes you can take at your local Y or gym; you can also purchase inexpensive weights at Sports Authority or another sporting goods store. There is a wide selection of DVDs that will help you get the moves just right.

One don't: Avoid exercising right before you go to sleep. Because this will energize you, your sleep cycle may be affected. Schedule your exercise at least four hours before you go to bed.

• METABOLIC SYNDROME: THE BIPOLAR RISK

Unfortunately, when weight increases, so does the risk for metabolic syndrome—a cluster of risk factors that are associated with cardiovascular disease. These risk factors include diabetes, high LDL cholesterol (the "bad" one that clogs up your artery walls), increased visceral fat (fat cells that settle in your waist and abdominal areas), and high blood pressure. In fact, in one study of both schizophrenic and bipolar patients, 42.4 percent met the criteria for metabolic syndrome.[9]

But all is not lost. These conditions are all treatable, and under a physician's supervision, you should be able to lower your cholesterol and your blood pressure. And you can prevent *more* weight gain by eating healthful foods and exercising.

Relax

Stress is a fact of life. It's the way we cope with it that counts. If you have bipolar II, stress can be particularly risky. Too much and you could wind up hypomanic or manic. Stress can also make you so out of sorts that you get depressed. How do *you* handle stress?

Take the "Stress Test" in Figure 11-1 and see whether you have it under control.

FIGURE 11-1. Stress Test

Look over the following statements and see whether any of them pertain to you. If more than three ring true, your stress could be dangerously close to making you manic. Seek help from a health care professional to reduce your stress.

1. There always seems to be a deadline at work that I'm rushing to meet.
2. I'll start watching some TV or read a page-turner, and before I know it, it's two in the morning.
3. My work buddies like to go out for a drink after work, and they always ask me to join them.
4. My friends are always telling me how I can improve: my clothes, my significant other, my career.
5. My friends tell me I don't need meds or therapy.
6. My significant other is unavailable—either working late or being distant.
7. I use a lot of sugar in my coffee.
8. I can't sleep.
9. I'm so tired from the work week that I end up sleeping all day Saturday.
10. I'm really losing money on my gym membership. I hardly ever go.
11. I love sweets.
12. My boss is always criticizing me.
13. I have to work in a cubicle and hear every word others are saying. It's very distracting.
14. There's a work colleague who's in competition with me.
15. I haven't had any sex for a long time. It's just as well—I'm too wired.
16. I can't remember the last time I laughed.

continues

17. My heart is always racing and I'm always saying two things at once.
18. I have a "to do" list that's a mile long.
19. I haven't been out with my friends for a while. I want to be alone.
20. I feel like my illness has short-changed me—but I absolutely refuse to think about it!
21. I feel depressed, but I'm trying to fight it.
22. I've just had a traumatic event: a divorce, a new job, a move, a marriage.

There are several ways to deal with stress. Here are some coping techniques that many people with bipolar disorder successfully use to keep calm.

Find a work life that fits. For some of us that means self-employment. For others, it means a job that is fairly routine. If the work you love is fast-paced (or you have no financial choice), make sure what you do at work stays at work. Keep to a personal routine that gives you enough sleep and down time; stay away from caffeine and sugar.

Get a massage. There's nothing quite as relaxing as someone working on your tense muscles in a room lit by candlelight, with soothing music playing softly in the background and the scent of a calming oil, like lavender, in the air. The good news today is that massage can be affordable to most people. Health insurance companies offer discounts, and there are even massage "chains," such as Massage Envy, that offer less-expensive options.

Take a hot bath. Fill it with skin-softening oils or lavender bubbles. Sink slowly into it. Don't like baths? Use a relaxing-formula body shampoo in the shower.

Surround yourself with supportive people. I remember a psychiatrist whose book I was helping to write who told me that you are who you are with. If you are around negative people, you'll feel negative. If you are around understanding, positive people, you'll feel great. Of course, sometimes shedding destructive relationships is easier said than done. Talk to your therapist about ways to handle them that won't add to your stress.

Keep to your routine. You can't go wrong if you've created a realistic schedule that works for you. The key phrase: *that works for you.* You'll achieve a sense of control, which will make you calmer.

Try yoga. There's nothing like a good stretch to ease your aching back and float away your stress. There are several types of yoga that are explicitly meant to help you relax:

- *Integral yoga* follows a strict set of poses; it's nonstrenuous and very routine—and relaxing. It's the one I prefer.
- *Kundalini yoga* allows you to move the way you want; if you feel more relaxed with your arm in front of you instead of in back, go for it. Using props, such as straps or blocks, to help with the poses is encouraged.
- *Restorative yoga* is designed to soothe. It's particularly rejuvenating for people who are recovering from an illness, who have a chronic condition (such as bipolar II), who are overweight, or who simply need to reduce their stress levels.

Meditate. Some people believe that if they don't get to meditate for at least ten minutes when they wake up, they'll be too stressed to deal with their day—and these are people *without* bipolar II. Meditation gives you a sense of calm and peace. You'll be energized but not hyper; you'll feel centered.

There really isn't a great mystery about meditation, and anyone can do it. You can either sit up or lie down on your back. You can repeat a word over and over (many people use the universal "Om" sound, which is supposed to ground you). You can stare at a lit candle until you have to close your eyes. (Just make sure your candle is in an open area with plenty of wick.) You can use a strand of beads (sold in health food stores), counting each one as it passes through your fingers. You can use a CD or DVD specially produced for guided meditation and creative visualization; just close your eyes and listen. You can pray. (However, Holly Swartz, M.D., recommends staying away from meditation if you are in the throes of a deep depression; the stillness can pull you down further.[10])

Accept your condition. Mourn for the life you can't have because of your bipolar II; grieve, cry, bang on the walls, and yell at your therapist. And then . . . release. A tremendous weight will be lifted from your shoulders. Acceptance brings peace.

Take a walk. It's a beautiful day, the sun is shining. Why not put on a pair of walking shoes or sneakers and stroll around the neighborhood. Not only will you be helping yourself relax, but you'll also be helping your heart.

• WHAT TO DO WHEN A HYPOMANIC EPISODE FEELS IMMINENT

Just like someone who's had too much to drink, a person who's beginning to feel that elated, impulsive, I-can-do-anything feeling needs his or her "designated driver." Here are some suggestions to keep the high from hitting the sky.

- Give your car keys and credit cards to a trusted companion.
- Make sure you stick to your routine—deciding in *advance* how late you'll be staying out.
- Avoid alcohol and other substances.
- Minimize your contact with confrontational people. If that means calling in sick to work, so be it.
- Take your medication religiously.
- Call your psychiatrist to see whether you should make any modifications to your regimen.

• A DEEP-BREATHING EXERCISE TO HELP YOU SLEEP

1. Lie down on your bed, face up, arms and legs outstretched (but relaxed). Put the covers around you and get comfortable.
2. Take a deep breath. Hold it. Count to 8. Breathe out. Count to 8.
3. Repeat this deep breathing three times.
4. Clench your toes, then release.
5. Flex your calves, then release.
6. Flex your thighs, then release.
7. Contract your stomach, then release.
8. Clench your fingers, then release.
9. Clench your lower arms, then release.
10. Flex your upper arms, then release.
11. Wrinkle up your face, open your mouth, and stick out your tongue.
12. Release.
13. Breathe gently in and out.
14. Good night!

Bipolar and the Real World

There's a scene in an old movie that takes place in a Bloomingdale's bedding department. The actress Jill Clayburgh is having an anxiety attack, and the man with her (Burt Reynolds—I told you this was an old movie) shouts out, "Does anyone have a Valium?!" A crowd gathers, shouting, "I do! I do!" the joke being that *everyone* takes Valium because they need to calm down.

That is actually far from the truth. Today, psychotropic medications have gotten a bum rap. People are writing and reading and appearing on TV to say how antidepressants can make you feel worse, how entirely too many pills are being popped, how you don't need pills or a therapist. All you need is some life-coaching and some discipline.

So where does that leave someone with bipolar II (especially someone, like me, who's tried the coaching and the strict routine to no avail)? Unfortunately, where it leaves such a person is usually in the closet. I'll be honest: I was afraid of writing this book and letting the world know that I have this disorder. I was afraid of the disapproval or shock of those I've known, those I've worked with, those I haven't told.

Let's face it. No one wants to lose their job. No one wants their significant other to walk away. And bipolar disorder, in most circles, still means it's only a matter of time before you take the stapler from your desk and staple everyone within reach, or you're going to start screaming in a restaurant, waving a fork, or you'll wind up alone, in bed, dying from the loss of blood from the ear you just cut off.

Is it really that way? Read the letter in Figure 11-2, which Randy Cohen kindly let me reprint from his *The Ethicist* column in the *New York Times Magazine*.

The good news is that there are people like Randy Cohen—more and more each day—who realize that mental illness isn't something you need be afraid of.

The real world is just that: full of swirling contradictions, changing views, accepting and rejecting. All I can do is offer some hints from the experts on what you should do . . . and when.

Going to Work

A whopping 88 percent of people with depression and bipolar disorder say that their condition hurt their careers.[11] But that is more a reflection on the stress of trying to hide the disorder, or of being in a job that doesn't work for you, than on your ability to do the job.

FIGURE 11-2. A letter to Randy Cohen, The Ethicist Columnist, and His Response from *The New York Times Magazine*, June 24, 2007

My nanny recently told me that she takes antipsychotic medication for a bipolar disorder. I've been happy with her for the past two years. She seldom spends long hours alone with my children because I am a stay-at-home mother, and she would never knowingly harm them, but people with psychosis can't always control themselves. You don't fire someone for a disability, and I feel a particular sense of obligation because she is a young undocumented Haitian, but should I dismiss her to protect my children?

You should not fire your nanny. Your anxiety stems more from lurid notions of mental illness—"Psycho" and "The Snake Pit" are not documentaries—than any real risk to your children. Your nanny has never endangered them; you've long admired her work.

You are restrained not only by ethics but also by the spirit of the Americans with Disabilities Act. An attorney I consulted says that if you ran a larger business, "to fire her would be illegal." Were she to stop taking her medication or otherwise display dangerous behavior, a business could dismiss her. Fortunately, as a stay-at-home mother, you can see if her condition deteriorates before anyone is imperiled.

Her immigration status already restricts her other employment prospects, and her limited options, as you imply, impose an additional ethical burden on you. If she can do the job, she should be allowed to keep it.

Remember, you don't have to tell anyone about your condition. Your health is your business—only. But if your bipolar II is affecting your performance, it might be a good idea to tell your boss and your colleagues. They'll better understand the changes in your behavior and, one can hope, be more understanding. But before you tell:

Determine what you want from your job—and the benefits of "coming out." Do you want shorter hours? Do you want less responsibility? Do you need a vacation? Ask yourself whether this is the job you want.

Go over your finances. See if you can afford to take time off. Make a budget to see what you really need to live on until you can find a job better suited for you. Check into your firm's disability insurance policy. Talk to your therapist about the Family and Medical Leave Act and Social Security Disability Insurance. Would pursuing these help you stay on your feet?

Take time to really think about it. People with bipolar disorder can act impulsively. Make sure this is a sound decision; talk to your family and your friends before saying, "I quit."

Talking to Your Family and Friends

Bipolar disorder can put a tremendous strain on all your relationships, especially that with your significant other. But you need your loved ones' support, and telling people who are close to you will help you in the long run. Consider:

Joining a support group and hearing what other people with the same condition have done when it came to telling their loved ones. You can find support groups in your area by checking the Depression and Bipolar Support Alliance (DBSA) website, www.DBSAlliance.org, or through your therapist or local hospital.

Asking your family to come to therapy with you or beginning family-focused therapy (FFT) so that the whole family is "on the same page." (See Chapter 10 for information on FFT.)

Educating your loved ones. Give them booklets and brochures from such organizations as the DBSA. You can download information or have booklets on a variety of bipolar subjects mailed to you.

Enlisting their help. Your loved ones will probably see the signs of an episode brewing before you do. They can help you stick to your routine and your medications, and if the need arises, they can call your psychiatrist or psychotherapist for help.

Listening. Bipolar disorder isn't easy on anyone. Let your family and friends discuss how they felt during one of your depressions, or how they might have looked on helplessly as you rushed through all your chores, finished all your work, bought all the skin care items on QVC, and couldn't sleep a wink.

Reaching out. When you were depressed, you may have pushed the world away, not wanting to see anyone. But isolation will only make things worse. Push yourself to call your friends; make a date (and put it on your schedule). The same goes for your mania. If you've embarrassed or angered someone you love when you were manically anxious, don't hide. Chances are that if someone loves you, she or he will love you through thick and thin—or, in this case, through depression and mania.

A healthy lifestyle works for everyone. But if you have bipolar II, it takes on extra meaning. Taking care of yourself, staying healthy, and learning relaxation techniques not only keep your body and mind in balance but can also stave off many of the more dramatic symptoms of bipolar II: debilitating anxiety, irritability, inappropriate extravagance, and anger.

12

Bipolar II and Creativity

Creativity represents a miraculous coming together of the uninhibited energy of the child with its apparent opposite and enemy, the sense of order imposed on the disciplined adult intelligence.

—Norman Podhoretz

CREATIVITY. THE WORD alone provokes mystery and adventure: the artist writing or painting masterpieces in a Parisian garret; the poet sitting beneath a tree, capturing the nature of things in verse; a Greek muse offering inspiration; a driven writer perched on the bed late at night, banging out the next best seller on a laptop.

Whatever visuals you imagine when you think about creativity —toss them out. Taking medication to treat your bipolar II will not "destroy" your creative side. If anything, it can help you focus on the creative task at hand; the medication can actually help you finish it.

We might get a spark when we're hypomanic, but the true test of creativity is being able to organize the work of art, to put it down on paper or easel or stone so that it makes sense. As Thomas Edison famously said, "Creativity is 10 percent inspiration and 90 percent perspiration." If you are anxious, hyper, wired, or overly confident, you're not going to get the results you want—no matter how talented you are. Don't use the belief that your talent will disappear as an excuse to stop taking your meds. You will still be you when you stick to your medication regimen—but a happier, easier you.

Creativity + Artistic Talent = Bipolar Disorder?

Nancy C. Andreasen, M.D., University of Iowa College of Medicine, was the first psychiatrist to use clinical criteria to explore the relationship between creativity and mental disorders. In 1970, she matched thirty of the writers at the prestigious University of Iowa Writers' Workshop with thirty people of exactly the same age, education, and gender, but with no interest in "the arts." The result? Ten of the writers had mood disorders, compared with only two in the control group. And only two of those ten writers had classic manic-depression. The majority had mood swings with milder mania and/or hypomania, which, as we know today, is most likely bipolar II.[1]

In her book *Touched by Fire: Manic Depressive Illness and the Artistic Temperament*, Kay Redfield Jamison, Ph.D., the scientist and author who wrote the classic memoir about her own bipolar disorder in *An Unquiet Mind*, demonstrates that, unfortunately, artistic temperament and bipolar disorder seem to go hand in hand.[2]

Dr. Jamison also conducted a survey on the possible mood swings of the most famous forty-seven British authors and writ-

• FAMOUS PEOPLE WITH BIPOLAR DISORDER

Carrie Fisher
Maurice Bernard (Emmy-winning actor on *General Hospital*)
Rosemary Clooney
Moss Hart (award-winning playwright and biographer)
Vivian Leigh
Ben Stiller
Robert Downey, Jr.
Sylvia Plath
Vincent Van Gogh
Robin Williams
Lili Taylor
Alvin Ailey
Joshua Logan (famous Broadway director and producer)
Gustave Mahler
Ted Turner
Buzz Aldrin
Ludwig von Beethoven
Ernest Hemingway
Sting
Tom Waits
Hart Crane
Robert Lowell
Jane Pauley
Virginia Woolf
General George S. Patton
Kay Redfield Jamison (author and scientist)
Teddy Roosevelt

And the list goes on. . . .

ers. It turned out that 38 percent of them—or thirty times more than the percentage in the general population—had indeed sought treatment for mood swings. Poets and novelists were the most often affected; half of them needed psychiatric treatment (drugs and/or hospitalization); two-thirds of the playwrights she interviewed sought treatment (mainly psychotherapy); and 13 percent of fine artists had sought help.[3]

Think about the creative connection. People in the throes of creative exuberance, as Dr. Jamison calls it, are usually

Highly sensitive to their world. Creative people observe things that others overlook; they can feel things more strongly; they can express themselves in ways that are unique—and creative.

Less inhibited. Because they "let the outside in," creative people are more prone to make original, albeit sometimes far-fetched, connections; they are more willing to step inside their unconscious. Their thoughts flow fast and furious.

Extremely focused. Creative people, once on the creative path, can focus so intently on the project at hand that all else is excluded. They can fully concentrate on their novel, their poem, their art: they may create at a fever pitch.

Sounds a lot like hypomania, doesn't it? And, let's face it, you don't have to be a creative genius to love that always-too-brief period. Who wouldn't like a chance to be hypomanic? You feel more alive. You can accomplish much more. You're bursting with ideas, and everyone wants to be with you. But then—and here's the difference between creative energy and bipolar hypomania—comes the fall. Either you sink into an anxiety-ridden, tortuous mania in which you're frozen, or you suddenly spiral down into the depression you left for that "one bright, shining moment."

A Healthy Creativity

Ernest Hemingway once said, "Never mistake motion for action." The frantic pace, the frenetic thoughts, the fear and anxiety of bipolar II mania aren't going to help you write that novel or paint a still life. In fact, a 2004 study that examined the research on creativity and bipolar disorder found that the connection was vastly overstated.[4] The elements of creativity do resemble hypomania, but that could be "the creativity talking," not the disease. It is also possible that creativity and bipolar disorder *share* some of the same genes—but are not exactly the same.[5]

So what do you do? Free your creative potential or treat a serious disease? Fire up your imagination or have a substandard quality of life?

Elizabeth was terrified that the mood stabilizers her doctor prescribed for her bipolar II would destroy her ability to paint. To her, being an artist was to be half-mad. In her mind, she was living the "artist in the garret" fantasy; she was Monet or Renoir or even Van Gogh.

Elizabeth decided not to take her meds, and her illness grew worse. She became agoraphobic; she lost her circle of friends. Her husband left her. She thought about suicide. During this painful time, Elizabeth continued to paint; she worked all night and watched the sun come up. She smoked cigarette after cigarette in her San Francisco loft and played her iPod at full volume. And, just as in the movies, a gallery owner saw her work and asked her to do a one-woman show.

It was a dream come true! Elizabeth started putting together her canvases. But every time she decided which ones to show, she changed her mind. She couldn't decide. She went to bed, paralyzed with anxiety. She made excuse after excuse until the gallery owner stopped calling. Elizabeth never got to do her show. She might have had the "fire in the belly," but no one else would ever know. Would she have been able to do work of the same quality if she'd taken medicine?

Some experts say yes. The medicines for bipolar II are mild compared to those prescribed for other illnesses, including bipolar I; the dosages are smaller. If anything, treatment would have eased the anxiety enough for Elizabeth to organize her show.

Still other experts say no, that the medicines may indeed stifle creativity.

Which view is correct?

I know that for me, the answer was and continues to be clear: take the medicine and run. Ironically, before I was diagnosed, those pearls of imagination, those rhythmic, cryptic explosions of words, were just that: small kernels and snippets. I'd never have been able to write this book from start to finish. Nor would I have been able to start a novel the first few chapters of which got me a scholarship to a writers' retreat in Vermont in 2008. A whole month just to write!

Before I was diagnosed, I'd never have been able to get far enough along to submit *any* pages of a novel for a writers' retreat. And if I somehow *did* get that far, I'd never have been able to take advantage of the opportunity. I'd be wondering what was lurking outside my cabin. I'd be wondering who liked me and who ignored me at dinner. I'd be writing nothing but those self-defeating but familiar "Who am I trying to kid?" love notes to myself.

But today, because I take care of myself (most of the time), go to a psychotherapist (once a week), and take my medications (religiously), I am able actually be the full creative being I wanted to be forty some years ago.

I remember a writing teacher I had a long time ago. On the very first day of class, he told everyone to make sure they didn't sacrifice their lives for their art. "What if you don't become famous? What then?" he said. "You'll have nothing."

Put another way, when it comes to creativity and bipolar disorder, you need to nourish yourself first. Take your medications, get help, and improve your quality of life—the creativity will flow even better! I'll take treatment every time. I believe in feeding the fire, but putting out the flames.

• THE CREATIVE FIRE

Fortunately, it isn't an either-or situation. You can have your creativity—and your medications, too. Here are some suggestions from the painters, writers, and sculptors I interviewed for this book.

- *Play music that is deeply personal* and moving to you. Whether a Beethoven symphony or a Beatles song, it can keep you inspired.
- *Use creative visualization techniques.* Imagine yourself finished with a project, how satisfied and proud you feel, how exhilarated. See your project come to life—and you will be that much closer to the reality.
- *Read an inspiring book about creativity* and art, such as Julia Cameron's *The Artist's Way*. An instructive, positive book about your art keeps you optimistic about your goal—and ensures that your creativity is nourished.
- *Keep a journal.* Ideas blossom as you write. If you write a few pages in a notebook every morning, you'll not only start brimming with ideas—you'll be calmer to boot.
- *Go to a museum.* Feed your soul by walking through the sound-absorbing corridors, seeing great works of art from the past, artifacts from ancient civilizations, creatures from the sea or land. Wander, stop, look.

Epilogue
Life as a Swimming Pool

TODAY, FIVE YEARS after I was correctly diagnosed with bipolar II, I am infinitesimally aware of my moods. Despite the fact that I finally have a correct diagnosis and I'm getting the treatment I need, it's still a delicate balancing act. I still have trouble differentiating my mania from my depression, it's that subtle. In the midst of a depression, I may feel an intense anxiety that borders on mania. In the midst of a good cycle, where I feel more focused and enthusiastic, I may have a niggling pang that it's not real; it's really nervous energy, the "feel good" hypomania before the anxiety, fear, and hypervigilance that mark my bipolar II mania. I'll buy a pair of shoes and worry that I'm entering a spending spiral. I'll wonder why I haven't heard from a friend in a while and worry that a cycle of anxiety is beginning.

I'm highly sensitive to the medication I take. The slightest bit too much of my anticonvulsant, and I'll plunge into a dire depression within hours. The slightest bit too little and I'll start feeling the old, familiar nervous energy. I now know what people mean when they say they "eat" a pill. I will literally nibble my

Seroquel when I'm nervous in order to strike the perfect balance between calmness and focus.

And there is always the possibility that the combination of drugs I'm currently taking will suddenly stop working; I'll have to change the dosage or the drug itself. Studies show that long-term effects on the brain are highly variable. Stress, hormonal change, physical illness—all these can affect the way the body metabolizes a medication. Like a car that requires proper maintenance, I have to go to my psychiatrist every few months for a "tune up" to make sure I'm stable.

Regret is a problem as well, a bittersweet pill. On occasion, I miss my "bigger than life" hypomania moments and feel tempted to flush my medication down the toilet. And I get tired of my own particular set of side effects, especially the weight gain.

But I always remember what it was like before I was properly diagnosed. I realize that I'm much more comfortable in my skin, and I'll keep taking my pills with the morning paper, keep going to my weekly psychotherapy appointments, and keep buying clothes that fit no matter what the size.

The people I've interviewed for this book are in similar places. After years of misdiagnosis, they finally have a name for their pain. And they, too, have to watch themselves and wonder whether they are getting a little too wired or a little too sad.

If nothing else, I hope this book brings more attention to bipolar II, a condition that affects so many millions of Americans. And I hope it helps you find an answer to your pain before another year goes by.

I remember an afternoon about a year ago. I was walking in the park with my husband and dogs. We were talking; the breezes were rustling the trees; the sun was bright. I laughed at something and it hit me: I hadn't worried. I hadn't been hyper-vigilant. I was in the moment having fun.

It was an amazing feeling, one that you can feel as well with the right treatment.

And if you are currently undergoing treatment, I hope, too, that this book has helped you learn, as we all did, that you have to keep the chemicals in that swimming pool in perfect balance, checking the levels every day. But once you do, the water is crystal clear, the pool is clean, and the swimming is magnificent.

May you too find the water just right, the sky sparkling, and your world at peace.

Appendix A
Weekly Schedule

TIME	MONDAY	TUESDAY	WEDNESDAY	THURSDAY	FRIDAY	SATURDAY	SUNDAY
5–6 A.M.							
6–7 A.M.							
7–8 A.M.							
8–9 A.M.							
9–10 A.M.							
10–11 A.M.							
11–noon							
noon–1 P.M.							

TIME	MONDAY	TUESDAY	WEDNESDAY	THURSDAY	FRIDAY	SATURDAY	SUNDAY
1–2 P.M.							
2–3 P.M.							
3–4 P.M.							
4–5 P.M.							
5–6 P.M.							
6–7 P.M.							
7–8 P.M.							

TIME	MONDAY	TUESDAY	WEDNESDAY	THURSDAY	FRIDAY	SATURDAY	SUNDAY
8–9 P.M.							
9–10 P.M.							
10–11 P.M.							
11–midnight							
midnight–1 A.M.							
1 A.M.–2 A.M.							
2 A.M.–3 A.M.							
3 A.M.–4 A.M.							

Appendix B
Resources

I've compiled a list of resources that I found helpful both in my research and for myself. Each of these sites provides information on bipolar disorder; many of them offer brochures you can download or have mailed to you. Some of the sites have e-newsletters about bipolar that you can subscribe to. Some of these are also opinions from people who have suffered from bipolar disorder; their blogs and websites are also mentioned here.

I have not included the sites of the pharmaceutical companies that manufacture the different medications, because their information may be more biased.

BipolarConnect.com: Share Your Experience: Postings
www.healthcentral.com/bipolar

Bipolar World
www.bipolarworld.net

Centers for Disease Control and Prevention (CDC)
www.cdc.gov

Childhood and Adolescent Bipolar Foundation
www.bpkids.org

Consumer Reports Best Buy Drugs
www.crbestbuydrugs.org

Depression and Bipolar Support Alliance
www.DBSAlliance.com

Depression Fallout by Anne Sheffield
www.depressionfallout.com

Dr. Deb: A Blog
http://drdeborahserani.blogspot.com

HealthCentral.com
www.healthcentral.com

The Juvenile Bipolar Research Foundation
www.jbrf.org

KidsHealth for Kids: The Nemours Foundation
kidshealth.org/kid/health_problems/learning_problem/bipolar_disorder

Living with a Purple Dog: The Ramblings of a Bipolar Product of the Seventies: G. J. "Jon" Gregory
http://livingbipolar.blogspot.com

McMan's Depression and Bipolar Web
www.mcmanweb.com

The Mayo Foundation for Medical Education and Research
www.mayoclinic.com

Medline
www.nlm.nih.gov/medlineplus

Mental Health America
www.nhma.org

Mood Garden
www.moodgarden.org

National Alliance on Mental Illness
www.nami.org

National Institute on Disability and Rehabilitation Research
www.ed.gov/about/offices/list/osers/nidrr

National Institutes of Health
www.nih.gov

National Institute of Mental Health
www.nimh.nih.gov

Pendulum.org
www.pendulum.org

PsychEducation.org
http://psycheducation.org

PubMed: A Service of the National Library of Medicine and the National Institutes of Health
www.ncbi.nl.mnih.gov/sites

Social Security Administration
www.ssa.gov

Substance Abuse and Mental Health Services Administration
www.mentalhealth.samhsa.gov

The Trouble with Spikol: A Blog about Mental Health
http://trouble.philadelphiaweekly.com

U.S. Food and Drug Administration
www.fda.gov

Wing of Madness
www.wingofmadness.com/index.php

Notes

Foreword

1. Altamura AC, Mundo E, Dell'Osso B, et al. Quetiapine and classical mood stabilizers in the long-term treatment of bipolar disorder: a 4-year follow-up naturalistic study. *J Affect Disord.* 2008: Epub ahead of print: March 8.

Introduction

1. Hirschfeld RMA, Calabrese JR, Weissman MM, et al. Screening for bipolar disorder in the community. *J Clin Psychiatry.* 2003; 64: 53–59.
2. *Living with Bipolar Disorder: How Far Have We Really Come?* National Depressive and Manic-Depressive Association (NDMDA) Constituency Survey, 2001.

1. A Disease in Its Own Right

1. Judd LL, Akiskal HS, Schettler PJ, et al. The comparative clinical phenotype and long term longitudinal episode course of bipolar I and II: a clinical spectrum or distinct disorders? *J Affect Disord.* 2003; 73: 19–32.
2. Perugi G, Akiskal HS. The soft bipolar spectrum redefined: focus on the cyclothymic, anxious-sensitive, impulse-dyscontrol, and binge-eating connection in bipolar II and related conditions. *Psychiatr Clin N Am.* 2002; 25: 713–737.

3. Perugi G, Toni C, Tavierso M. The role of cyclothymia in atypical depression: toward a data-based reconceptualization of the borderline-bipolar II connection. *J Affect Disord.* 2003; 73: 87–98.

4. Akiskal HS. Classification, diagnosis, and boundaries of bipolar disorders. In: Maj M, Akiskal HS, Lopez-Ibor JJ, Sartorius N, eds. *Bipolar Disorder, Vol. 5.* West Sussex, United Kingdom: John Wiley & Sons; 2002: 1–52.

5. Rihmer Z, Pestality P. Bipolar II disorder and suicidal behavior. *Psychiatr Clin N Am.* 1999; 22: 667–673.

6. Judd LL, Akiskal HS, Schettler PJ, et al. The comparative clinical phenotype and long term longitudinal episode course of bipolar I and II: a clinical spectrum or distinct disorders? *J Affect Disord.* 2003; 73: 19–32.

7. Angst J. The emerging epidemiology of hypomania and bipolar II disorder. *J Affect Disord.* 1998; 50: 143–151.

8. Ten HM, Vollebergh W, Bijl R, et al. Bipolar disorder in the general population in The Netherlands (prevalence, consequences, and care utilization): results from The Netherlands Mental Health Survey and Incidence Study (NEMESIS). *J Affect Disord.* 2002; 68: 203–213.

9. American Psychiatric Association. *Diagnostic and Statistical Manual for Mental Disorders,* Fourth Edition, Text Revision. Washington, DC: American Psychiatric Association; 2000.

10. Leibenluft E. Issues in the treatment of women with bipolar illness. *J Clin Psychiatry.* 1997; 58 (suppl 15): 5S–11S.

11. Angst J. The emerging epidemiology of hypomania and bipolar II disorder. *J Affect Disord.* 1998; 50: 143–151.

12. Akiskal HS. The depressive phase of bipolar disorder: focus on bipolar II. Paper presented at 154th Annual Meeting of the American Psychiatric Association; May 2001: New Orleans, LA.

13. Marangell, LB. In discussion with Kupfer DJ, Sachs GS, et al. Emerging therapies for bipolar depression. February 9, 2006. Highlights presented in *J Clin Psychiatry.* 2006; 67: 7.

2. Hypomania Defined

1. Jamison KR. *Exuberance: The Passion for Life.* New York: Knopf; 2004.

2. McManamy J. *Living Well with Depression and Bipolar: What Your Doctor Doesn't Tell You That You Need to Know.* New York: Collins; 2006.

3. Angst J, Adolfsson R, Benazzi F, et al. The HCL-32: Towards a self-assessment tool for hypomanic symptoms in outpatients. *J Affect Disord.* 2005; 88: 217–233.

4. McManamy J. Special Hypomania Issue. *McMan's depression and bipolar weekly* 2005; 7 (10). http://www.mcmannweb.com. Published May 14, 2005. Accessed May 15, 2005.

5. Gartner JD. *The Hypomanic Edge: The Link Between (a Little) Craziness and (a Lot of) Success in America.* New York: Simon and Schuster; 2005.

3. Swing High the Bipolar II Way: Anxiety

1. Hirschfeld RMA. Introduction: an overview of the issues surrounding the recognition and management of bipolar disorder and anxiety. *J Clin Psychiatry.* 2006; 67 (suppl 1): S3–S5.

2. Keller MB. Prevalence and impact of comorbid anxiety and bipolar disorder. *J Clin Psychiatry.* 2006; 67 (suppl 1): S5–S7.

3. Simon NM, Smoller JW, Fava M, et al. Panic disorder and bipolar disorder: anxiety sensitivity as a potential mediator of panic during manic states. *J Affect Disord.* 2005; 87: 101–105.

4. Hirschfeld RMA. Introduction: an overview of the issues surrounding the recognition and management of bipolar disorder and anxiety. *J Clin Psychiatry.* 2006; 67 (suppl 1): S3–S5.

5. Boylan KR, Bieling PJ, Marriott M, et al. Impact of comorbid anxiety disorders on outcome in a cohort of patients with bipolar disorder. *J Clin Psychiatry.* 2004; 65: 1106–1113.

6. National Institute of Mental Health. *Anxiety Disorders.* www.nimh.nih.gov/publicat/anxiety.cfm#anx2. Published 2006. Accessed June 19, 2007.

7. Boylan KR, Bieling PJ, Marriott M, et al. Impact of comorbid anxiety disorders on outcome in a cohort of patients with bipolar disorder. *J Clin Psychiatry* 2004; 65: 1106–1113.

8. National Institute of Mental Health. *Anxiety Disorders.* www.nimh.nih.gov/publicat/anxiety.cfm#anx2. Published 2006. Accessed June 19, 2007.

9. BC Partners for Mental Health and Addiction Information. *Obsessive-Compulsive Disorder.* www.heretohelp.bc.ca/publications/factsheets/ocd.shtml. Published 2003–2007. Accessed June 21, 2007.

10. National Institute of Mental Health. *Anxiety Disorders.* www.nimh.nih.gov/publicat/anxiety.cfm#anx2. Published 2006. Accessed June 19, 2007.

11. Stein MB, Torgrud LJ, Walker JR. Social phobia symptoms, subtypes and severity: findings from a community survey. *Arch Gen Psychiatry.* 2000; 57: 1046–1052.

12. Boylan KR, Bieling PJ, Marriott M, et al. Impact of comorbid anxiety disorders on outcome in a cohort of patients with bipolar disorder. *J Clin Psychiatry.* 2004; 65: 1106–1113.

13. National Institute of Mental Health. *Anxiety Disorders.* www.nimh.nih.gov/publicat/anxiety.cfm#anx2. Published 2006. Accessed June 19, 2007.

14. Davis JL. Is it really depression? Symptoms of depression, anxiety disorder and bipolar disorder have similarities—but require different treatments. Reviewed by: Nazario B. *WebMD.* Published 2007. http://www.webmd.com/anxiety-panic/guide/is-really-depression. Accessed June 8, 2007.

4. Swing Low the Bipolar II Way: Depression

1. Calabrese JR. Bipolar disorder: from childhood to adulthood. Paper presented at Harvard University Medical School Conference on Bipolar Disorder: From Childhood to Adulthood; November 2003: Cambridge, MA.

2. Akiskal, HS. The depressive phase of bipolar disorder: focus on bipolar II. 154th Annual Meeting of the American Psychiatric Association, May 5–10, 2001, New Orleans, LA.

3. West ED. Dally PJ. Effects of iproniazid in depressive syndromes. *Br Med J.* 1959; 1: 1491–1494.

4. Thase ME. Introduction: new directions in the treatment of atypical depression. *J Clin Psychiatry.* 2007; 68 (suppl 3).

5. Sullivan PF, Kessler RC, Kendler KS. Latent class analysis of lifetime depressive symptoms in the National Comorbidity Survey. *Am J Psychiatry.* 1998; 155: 1398–1406.

6. American Psychiatric Association. *Diagnostic and Statistical Manual for Mental Disorders,* Fourth Edition, Text Revision. Washington, DC: American Psychiatric Association; 2000.

7. Mental Health Net. Bipolar disorder: statistics and patterns. http://mentalhelp.net/poc/view_doc.php?type=doc&id=11200&cn=4. Published December 13, 2006. Accessed July 8, 2007.

8. Hirschfeld RM, Lewis L, Vornik LA. Perceptions and impact of bipolar disorder: how far have we really come? Results of the National Depressive and Manic-Depressive Association 2000 survey of individuals with bipolar disorder. *J Clin Psychiatry.* 2003; 64: 161–174.

9. Hantouche EG, Akiskal HS, Lancrenon S, et al. Systematic clinical methodology for validating a bipolar-II disorder: date in mid-stream from a French multi-site study (EPIDEP). *J Affect Disord.* 1998; 50: 163–173.

10. Post RM, Denicoff KD, Leverich GS, et al. Morbidity in 258 bipolar outpatients followed for 1 year with daily prospective ratings on the NIMH life chart method. *J Clin Psychiatry.* 2003; 64: 680–690.

11. Marangell, LB. In discussion with Kupfer DJ, Sachs GS, et al. Emerging therapies for bipolar depression. February 9, 2006. Highlights presented in *J Clin Psychiatry.* 2006; 67: 7.

5. The Bipolar Brain

1. Meeks, J. *High Times, Low Times: The Many Faces of Adolescent Depression.* New York: Bantam Books; 1988.

2. Schraer WD, Stoltze HJ. *Biology: A Comprehensive Text for New York State.* Newton, MA: Cebco; 1983: 50–69, 266–279.

3. Kluger J, Sora S. Young and bipolar. *Time Magazine.* August 19, 2002: 40–51.

4. Whybrow PC. *A Mood Apart. The Thinker's Guide to Emotion and Its Disorders.* New York: Harper Perennial; 1998.

5. Stein S. *The Body Book.* New York: Workman Publishing; 1992.

6. Kluger J, Sora S. Young and bipolar. *Time Magazine.* August 19, 2002: 40–51.

7. Neuroscience for Kids website. Available at: http://faculty.washington.edu/chudler/neurok.html. Accessed July 29, 2007.

8. Kluger J, Sora S. Young and bipolar. *Time Magazine*. August 19, 2002: 40–51.

9. Cassidy JW. *Brainstorms*. New York: Bantam Books; 1992.

10. Martin AR, Wallace BG, et al. *From Neuron to Brain: A Cellular and Molecular Approach to the Function of the Nervous System* (4th edition). Sunderland, MA: Sinauer Associates; 2001.

11. Zubieta J-K, Huguelet P, et al. High vesicular monoamine transporter binding in asymptomatic bipolar I disorder: sex differences and cognitive correlates. *Am J Psychiatry*. 2000; 157: 1619–1628.

12. Borodinsky LN, Root CM, et al. Activity-dependent homeostatic specification of transmitter expression in embryonic neurons. *Nature*. 2004; 429: 523–530.

13. Svenningsson P, Tzavara, ET, Liu F, et al. DARPP-32 mediates serotonergic neurotransmission in the forebrain. *PNAS*. 2002; 99 (5); 3188–3193.

14. Blakeslee S. Humanity? Maybe it's in the wiring. *New York Times*. December 9, 2003: F1–F4.

15. National Institutes of Mental Health. Available at: http://www.nimh.nih.gov. Accessed July 29, 2007.

16. Blakeslee S. Humanity? Maybe it's in the wiring. *New York Times*. December 9, 2003: F1–F4.

17. Ferszt R, Severus E, Bode L. Activated Borna disease virus in affective disorders. *Pharmacopsychiatry*. 1999; 32 (3): 93–98.

18. Kunzig R. It kills horses, doesn't it? *Discover*. October 1, 1997.

19. Ferszt R, Kuhl KP, Bode L. Amantadine revisited: an open trial of amantadine sulfate treatment in chronically depressed patients with Borna disease virus infection. *Pharmacopsychiatry*. 1999; 32(4):142–147.

6. Personality and Family History

1. McMahon FJ, Simpson SG, et al. Linkage of bipolar disorder to chromosone 18q and the validity of bipolar ii disorder. *Arch Gen Psychiatry*. 2001; 58: 1025–1031.

2. Baum AE, Akula N. A genome-wide association study implicates diacylglycerol kinase eta (DGKH) and several other genes in the etiology of bipolar disorder. *Molecular Psychiatry*. Advance online publication May 8, 2007; doi: 10.1038/sj.mp.4002012. Accessed August 1, 2007.

3. Stahl S. Molecular neurobiology for practicing physicians, part 3: how second messengers "turn on" genes by activating protein kinases and transcription factors. *J Clin Psychiatry.* 1999; 60.

4. Rihmer Z, Arato M. ABO blood groups in manic-depressive patients. *J Affect Disord.* 1981; 3: 1–7.

5. Depression and Bipolar Support Alliance (DBSA). www.dbsalliance.org. Accessed August 8, 2007.

6. Egeland JA, Shaw JA, Endicott J, et al. Prospective study of prodromal features for bipolarity in well Amish children. *J Am Acad Child Adolesc Psychiatry.* 2003; 42 (7): 786–796.

7. Dick DM, Foroud T, Flury L, et al. Genomewide linkage analyses of bipolar disorder: a new sample of 250 pedigrees from the National Institute of Mental Health genetics initiative. *Am J Hum Genet.* 2003; 73 (4): 979.

8. Chang K, Steiner H, Dienes K, et al. Bipolar offspring: a window into bipolar evolution. *Bio Psychiatry.* 2003; 53: 945–951.

9. Chess S, Thomas A. *Temperament in Clinical Practice.* Re-issue. New York: Guilford Press; 1995.

10. Chess S, Thomas A. Temperamental differences: a critical concept in child health care. *Pediatr Nurse.* 1985; 11 (3): 167–171.

11. Perugi G, Akiskal HS. The soft bipolar spectrum redefined: focus on the cyclothymic, anxious-sensitive, impulse-dyscontrol, and binge-eating connection in bipolar II and related conditions. *Psychiatr Clin North Am.* 2002; 25 (4): 713–737.

7. Diagnosis

1. Coryell W, Keller M, Endicott J, et al. Bipolar II illness: course and outcome over a five-year period. *Psychological Med.* 1989; 19:129–141.

2. Ghaemi SN, Sachs GS, Chiou AM, et al. Is bipolar disorder still underdiagnosed? Are antidepressants overutilized? *J Affect Disord.* 1999; 52: 135–144.

3. Akiskal HS. Switching from "unipolar" to bipolar II: an 11-year prospective study of clinical and temperamental predictors in 559 patients. *Arch Gen Psychiatry.* 1995; 52: 114–123.

4. Swartz HA. Telephone interview on August 9, 2007.

5. Benazzi F. Impulsivity in bipolar II disorder: trait, state, or both? *Euro Psychiatry.* 2007; 20· 1–7.

6. Benazzi F. Is overactivity the core feature of hypomania in bipolar II disorder? *Psychopathology.* 2007; 40: 54–60.

7. Keller, MB. Prevalence and impact of comorbid anxiety and bipolar disorder. *J Clin Psychiatry.* 2006; 67(1): 5–7.

8. Simon NM, Otto MW, Wisniewski SR, et al. Anxiety disorder comorbidity in bipolar disorder patients: data from the first 500 participants in the systematic treatment enhancement program for bipolar disorder (STEP-BD). *Am J Psychiatry.* December 2004; 161: 2222–2229.

9. Bowden CL. Strategies to reduce misdiagnosis of bipolar depression. *Psychiatric Serv.* January 2001; 52 (1): 51–54.

10. Senelick RC, Rossi P, Dougherty K. *Living with Stroke: A Guide for Families.* Revised Edition. Chicago: Contemporary Books; 1999.

11. Rihmer Z, Pestality P. Biopolar II disorder and suicidal behavior. *Psychiatr Clin North Am.* 1999; 22: 667–673.

12. Bowden CL. Strategies to reduce misdiagnosis of bipolar depression. *Psychiatric Serv.* 2001; 52 (1): 51–55.

13. Angst J, Adolfsson R, Benazzi F, et al. The HCL-32: towards a self-assessment tool for hypomanic symptoms in outpatients. *Jour Affect Disord.* 2005; 88: 217–233.

14. Pies R. Bipolar spectrum disorder scale (BSDS). Available at: http://www.psycheducation.org. Accessed August 26, 2007.

8. Pediatric Bipolar Disorder

1. Kluger, J, with Susan Song. Young and bipolar. *Time.* August 19, 2002.

2. Papolos D, Papolos J. *The Bipolar Child: The Definitive and Reassuring Guide to Childhood's Most Misunderstood Disorder.* Revised and expanded. New York: Broadway Books; 2002.

3. Papolos D, Papolos J. *The Bipolar Child: The Definitive and Reassuring Guide to Childhood's Most Misunderstood Disorder.* Revised and expanded. New York: Broadway Books; 2002.

4. McManamy, J. Special Demitri and Janice Papolos Bipolar Child Issue. *McMan's Depression and Bipolar Weekly.* 2004; 6 (25). http://www

.mcmannweb.com. Published October 20, 2004. Accessed September 23, 2007.

5. Papolos D, Papolos J. *The Bipolar Child: The Definitive and Reassuring Guide to Childhood's Most Misunderstood Disorder.* Revised and expanded. New York: Broadway Books; 2002.

6. McManamy, J. Special Demitri and Janice Papolos Bipolar Child Issue. *McMan's Depression and Bipolar Weekly.* 2004; 6 (25). http://www.mcmann web.com. Published October 20, 2004. Accessed September 23, 2007.

7. Cleveland Clinic Department of Psychiatry and Psychology. *Bipolar Disorder Guide: Children and Teens with Bipolar Disorder. WebMD.* http://www.webmd.com/bipolar-disorder/guide/bipolar-children-teens. Reviewed September 1, 2006. Accessed June 8, 2007.

8. Papolos D, Papolos J. *The Bipolar Child: The Definitive and Reassuring Guide to Childhood's Most Misunderstood Disorder.* Revised and expanded. New York: Broadway Books; 2002.

9. Wagner KD. Bipolar disorder and comorbid anxiety disorders in children and adolescents. *J Clin Psychiatry.* 2006; 67 (suppl 1): 16–20.

10. Hirschfeld RMA. An overview of the issues surrounding the recognition and management of bipolar disorder and comorbid anxiety. *J Clin Psychiatry.* 2006; 67 (suppl 1): 3–4.

11. Perlis RH, Miyahara S, Marangell LB, et al. Long-term implication of early onset in bipolar disorder: data from the first 1000 participants in the Systematic Treatment Enhancement Program for Bipolar Disorder (STEP-BD). *Biol Psychiatry.* 2004; 55: 875–881.

12. Masi G, Toni C, Perugi G, et al. Anxiety disorders in children and adolescents with bipolar disorder: a neglected comorbidity. *Can J Psychiatry.* 2001; 46: 797–802.

13. Masi G, Toni C, Perugi G, et al. Anxiety disorders in children and adolescents with bipolar disorder: a neglected comorbidity. *Can J Psychiatry.* 2001; 46: 797–802.

14. Masi G, Millepiedi S, Mucci M, et al. Generalized anxiety disorder in referred children and adolescents. *J Am Acad Child Adolesc Psychiatry.* 2004; 43: 752–760.

15. Masi G, Millepiedi S, Mucci M, et al. Generalized anxiety disorder in referred children and adolescents. *J Am Acad Child Adolesc Psychiatry.* 2004; 43: 752–760.

16. Biederman J, Faraone SV, Marrs A, et al. Panic disorder and agoraphobia in consecutively referred children and adolescents. *J Am Acad Child Adolesc Psychiatry.* 1997; 36: 214–223.

17. Biederman J, Faraone SV, Marrs A, et al. Panic disorder and agoraphobia in consecutively referred children and adolescents. *J Am Acad Child Adolesc Psychiatry.* 1997; 36: 214–223.

18. Jerrell JM, Shugart MA. Community-based care for youths with early and very early onset bipolar I disorder. *Bipolar Disord.* 2004; 6: 299–304.

19. Sood, AB, Weller E, Weller R. SSRIs in children and adolescents: where do we stand? *Current Psychiatry.* March 2004; 3(3): 83–89.

20. Wagner KD. Bipolar disorder and comorbid anxiety disorders in children and adolescents. *J Clin Psychiatry.* 2006; 67 (suppl 1): 16–20.

21. Papolos D, Papolos J. *The Bipolar Child: The Definitive and Reassuring Guide to Childhood's Most Misunderstood Disorder.* Revised and expanded. New York: Broadway Books; 2002.

9. Getting Help: Medications

1. Torrey EF, Knable MB. *Surviving Manic Depression: A Manual on Bipolar Disorder for Patients, Families and Providers.* New York: Basic Books; 2002.

2. Bipolar Disorder Health Center. *Bipolar Disorder: Lithium for Bipolar Disorder.* http://www.webmd.com/bipolar-disorder/bipolar-disorder-lithium. Accessed June 8, 2007.

3. Gutman DA, Gutman AR. *Emerging Therapies for Bipolar Disorder: A Clinical Update.* http://www.webmd.com/bipolar-disorder/advanced-reading-bipolar-new-meds?print=true. Accessed June 8, 2007.

4. Hirschfeld RMA. *How guidelines influence the treatment of bipolar depression.* Presented at the American Psychiatric Association 159th Annual Meeting; May 20–25, 2006; Toronto, Ontario, Canada.

5. Calabrese JR. *Key side effects of lamotrigine, olanzapine, and quetiapine: a session for the practicing psychiatrist.* Presented at the American Psychiatric Association 159th Annual Meeting; May 20–25, 2006; Toronto, Ontario, Canada.

6. Altamura AC. E-mail interview on July 4, 2007.

7. Perlis RH. The role of pharmacologic treatment guidelines for bipolar disorder. *J Clin Psychiatry.* 2005; 66 (suppl 3): 37–47.

8. Rihmer Z, Pestality P. Bipolar II disorder and suicidal behavior. *Psychiatr Clin North Am.* 1999; 22: 667–673.

9. Altamura AC. Treatment issues in bipolar II depression. *International Journal of Neuropsychopharmacology.* 2006; 9: 775–776.

10. Altamura AC. E-mail interview on July 4, 2007.

11. Fagiolini A. Is it really depression? *WebMD.* Available at: http://www.webmd.com/anxiety-panic/guide/is-really-depression. Accessed June 29, 2008.

12. Altamura AC. E-mail interview on October 25, 2007.

13. Bowden CL. Atypical antipsychotic augmentation of mood stabilizer therapy in bipolar disorder. *J Clin Psychiatry.* 2005; 66 (suppl 3): 12–19.

14. Keck PE, Jr, Straw JR, McElroy S. Pharmacologic treatment considerations in co-occuring bipolar and anxiety disorders. *J Clin Psychiatry.* 2006; 67 (suppl 1): 8–15.

15. Altamura AC. Bipolar spectrum and drug addiction. *J Affect Disord.* 2007; 99: 285.

16. Fagiolini A, Frank E, Scott JA, et al. Metabolic syndrome in bipolar disorder: findings from the Bipolar Disorder Center for Pennsylvania. *Bipolar Disord.* 2005; 7: 424–430.

17. McElroy SL, Frye MA, Suppes T, et al. Correlates of overweight and obesity in 644 patients with bipolar diosrder. *J Clin Psychiatry.* 2002; 63: 207–213.

18. Welch J. Interview on September 19, 2007.

10. Getting More Help: Therapies

1. Miklowitz DJ. A review of evidence-based psychosocial interventions for bipolar disorder. *J Clin Psychiatry.* 2006; 67 (suppl 1): 28–33.

2. Butzlaff RL, Hooley JM. Expressed emotion and psychiatric relapse: a meta-analysis. *Arch Gen Psychiatry.* 1998; 55: 547–552.

3. Bakalar N. Long-term therapy effective in bipolar depression. *New York Times.* April 10, 2007: F8.

4. Koukopoulos A. Ewald Hecker's description of cyclothymia as a cyclical mood disorder: its relevance to the modern concept of bipolar II. *J Affect Disord.* 2003; 73: 199–205.

5. Milkowitz DJ, Otto M, Frank E, et al. Psychosocial treatments for bipolar depression: a 1-year randomized trial from the Systematic Treatment Enhancement Program (STEP). *Arch Gen Psychiatry.* (in press).

6. Swartz H. Telephone interview on August 8, 2007.

7. Frank E, Kupfer DJ, Thase ME, et al. Inducing lifestyle regularity in recovering bipolar disorder patients: results from the maintenance therapies in bipolar disorder protocol. *Biol Psychiatry.* 1997; 41: 1165–1173.

8. Miklowitz DJ, Richards JA, George EL, et al. Integrated family and individual therapy for bipolar disorder: results of a treatment development study. *J Clin Psychiatry.* 2003; 64: 182–191.

9. Miklowitz DJ. A review of evidence-based psychosocial interventions for bipolar disorder. *J Clin Psychiatry.* 2006; 67 (suppl 11): 28–33.

10. Swartz H, Frank E, Frankel D. Interpersonal and social rhythm therapy for bipolar II disorder: treatment development and case examples. *Revue de Santé Mentale au Québec* (in press).

11. Thase ME. Advanced reading: bipolar disorder psychotherapy. htttp://www/webmd/com/bipolar-disorder/guide/advanced-reading-bipolar-psychotherapy?print=true. Accessed June 8, 2007.

12. Scott J, Paykel E, Morriss R, et al. Cognitive behaviour therapy for bipolar. *Br J Psychiatry.* 2006; 188: 488–489.

13. Sachs GS. Strategies for improving treatment of bipolar disorder: integration of measurement and management. *Acta Psychiatrica Scand.* 2004; 110 (suppl 422): 7–17.

14. Miklowitz DJ. A review of evidence-based psychosocial interventions for bipolar disorder. *J Clin Psychiatry.* 2006; 67 (suppl 11): 28–33.

15. Silverman T. The promise of supplements? *BP Magazine.* Fall 2007: 34–37.

16. Stoll AL, Severus E, Freeman M, et al. Omega-3 fatty acids in bipolar disorder: a preliminary double-blind, placebo-controlled trial. *Arch Gen Psychiatry.* 1999; 56: 407–412.

17. Health Center Red Flags. Natural bipolar remedy. *HealthyPlace.com.* Available at: http://www.healthyplace.com/communities/Bipolar/News _2007/treatment_alternative.asp Accessed June 29, 2008.

18. Ask the mental health expert: archives 2001–2004. *HealthierYou.com.* Available at: http://www.healthieryou.com/mhexpert/exp1122203d.html. Accessed June 29, 2008.

19. University of Texas Southwestern. Acupuncture for treatment of patients with bipolar disorder. About.com. Available at: http://www.mentalhealth.about.com/library/sci/0102blmanicpuncture0102.htm?p=1. Accessed June 29, 2008.

11. Living Well with Bipolar II: Making Healthy Choices

1. Why is sleep so important? *Depression and Bipolar Support Alliance.* http://www.dbsalliance.org/site/PageServer?pagename=about_sleep_why&printer_friendly=1. Accessed October 29, 2007.

2. Roybal K, Theobold D, Graham A, et al. Mania-like behavior induced by disruption of CLOCK. *Proc Natl Acad Sci USA.* 2007; 104 (15): 6406–6411.

3. Lei Y, Wang J, Klein PS, et al. Nuclear receptor rev-erbα is a critical lithium-sensitive component of the circadian clock. *Science.* 2006; 311 (5763): 1002–1005.

4. Healthy sleep tips. *National Sleep Foundation.* http://www.sleepfoundation.org/site/c.hulXKjM01xF/b.2419237/k.BCBO/Healthy_Sleep_Tips.htm Accessed October 28, 2007.

5. Kennedy R. Management of weight gain in bipolar disorder: a newsmaker interview with Joseph Calabrese, M.D. *Medscape Medical News.* http://www.medscape.com/viewarticle/461919_print. Published 2003. Accessed November 22, 2003.

6. Research in weight gain and bipolar disorder: an expert interview with Gary Sachs, M.D. *Medscape Psychiatry and Mental Health.* 2004; 9 (1). http://www.medscape.com/viewarticle/475416_print. Accessed October 29, 2007.

7. Otto MW, Church TS, Craft LL, et al. Exercise for mood and anxiety disorders. *J Clin Psychiatry.* 2007; 68 (5): 669–676.

8. Gaesser GA, Dougherty K. *The Spark: The Revolutionary 3-Week Fitness Plan That Changes Everything You Know about Exercise, Weight Control, and Health.* New York: Simon & Schuster; 2001.

9. Basu R, Brar JS, Chengappa KN, et al. The prevalence of the metabolic syndrome in patients with schizoaffective disorder—bipolar subtype. *Bipolar Disord.* 2004; 6: 314–318.

10. Swartz H, Frank E, Frankel D. Interpersonal and social rhythm therapy for bipolar II disorder: treatment development and case examples. *Revue de Santé Mentale au Québec* (in press).

11. Bipolar disorder and going to work. *WebMD*. http://www.webmd .com/bipolar-disorder/guide/going-to-work-bipolar?print=true. Published 2005. Accessed June 8, 2007.

12. Bipolar II and Creativity

1. Andreasen NC. Creativity and mental illness: prevalence rates in writers and their first-degree relatives. *Am J Psychiatry*. 1987; 144:1288–1292.

2. Jamison KR. *Touched by Fire: Manic Depressive Illness and the Artistic Temperament*. New York: The Free Press 1996.

3. Holden C. Creativity and the troubled mind. *Psychology Today*. April 1987.

4. Janka Z. Artistic creativity and bipolar mood disorder. *Orv Hetil*. 2004; 145 (33): 1709–1718. (Original article in Hungarian.)

5. More evidence for link between mood disorders and creativity. *Stanford University Medical Center*. November 2005.

About the Author

KARLA DOUGHERTY has written forty-one books, including *Mindstorms: The Complete Guide for Families Living with Traumatic Brain Injury* (with John Cassidy, M.D.), *Chronic Fatigue for Dummies* (with Susan Lisman, M.D.), and *The Spark: The Revolutionary 3-Week Fitness Plan That Changes Everything You Know about Exercise, Weight Control, and Health* (with Glenn Gaesser, Ph.D.). She lives in Montclair, New Jersey.

Index